The Whartons'

stretch book

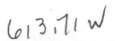

The Whartons'

stretch book

featuring
The Breakthrough Method of

Active-Isolated Stretching

Jim and Phil Wharton

with Bev Browning

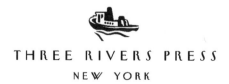

THREE RIVERS PRESS
NEW YORK

Copyright © 1996 by Jim & Phil Wharton and Maximum Performance International, Inc.

Published by Three Rivers Press, New York, New York.
Member of the Crown Publishing Group.

Random House, Inc. New York, Toronto, London, Sydney, Auckland
www.randomhouse.com

THREE RIVERS PRESS is a registered trademark and the Three Rivers Press colophon is a trademark of Random House, Inc.

Originally published by Times Books in 1996.

Printed in the United States of America

Book design by Publications Development Company

Library of Congress Cataloging-in-Publication Data is available upon request.

ISBN 0-8129-2623-4

15 14 13 12 11

To Aaron Mattes
Healer, Teacher, Mentor, and Friend

Acknowledgments

Special thanks and love to Michael Browning for lending Bev to us for a year and making us members of the family.

Thanks to Reid Boates, the world's greatest agent, and Elizabeth Rapoport, the world's greatest editor. Thanks so much for the generous efforts and talents of Ron Boyle, Ginna Frantz, Mike Weinstein, Terry Simes, Judith Laferriere, Diana Tonnessen, Sarah Bewley, Shannon Silcox, Vicki Poth, Angela St. Pierre, Randy Brower, and the athletes, clients and healthcare professionals who share our lives and our work every day.

JW
PW

Foreword

The Whartons' stretching program changed my life. Jim and Phil Wharton have reinvented what stretching is and what it can do for you.

When I ran the Lake Placid Sports Medicine Center, which was visited by top Olympians from around the world, I was always struck by how few athletes bothered to stretch. When I wrote my last book, *Turning Back the Clock,* I was tempted not to write a stretching chapter at all, because I couldn't find a program that really worked. Even though I've been a lifelong aerobic animal, competing in skiing, cycling, Iron Man contests, and marathons, neither I nor any of my friends ever stretched. Sure, we bought the books and tried a few of the exercises, but soon gave them up for lack of effect.

And then the Whartons introduced me to the next generation of stretching, called Active-Isolated Stretching (AI). Although scientists have been researching this for over twenty-five years and Olympians have been employing this technique for about eight years, AI stretching has only recently been brought to the public's attention, largely through the efforts of Jim and Phil Wharton. I had come to the Whartons believing that my hips were shot and that I needed major hip surgery. Then Jim took me through the hip flexion exercises. To my delight, he showed me that my hips were locked and could easily be unchained with AI stretching. This salvaged my flagging skiing, tennis, and blading career. I was astounded to realize increases of 40 degrees in my hip range of motion.

But the greatest strength of AI stretching is its ability to make a better athlete out of you. As we age, our muscles become increasingly inelastic. AI stretching can make substantial improvements in muscle elasticity, adding renewed life and spring to tired out old muscles. I'm faster and quicker now at 48 than I've ever been thanks to renewed muscle elasticity. But don't take my word for it. The real proof is in the Whartons' track record. The Whartons have trained thirty-three Olympians, eleven of whom have medaled. After Wharton worked with Dennis Mitchell, the 1992 bronze medalist in the 100 meter, for just a year, his time dropped from 10.03 seconds to 9.91. Phil Wharton told me, "In specific athletes, we've gotten an extra foot on the long jump and triple jump." Deep muscle stretching has allowed Olympic skier Alberto Tomba to transform his incredible strength into explosive power.

The Whartons' program also helps prevent injury. I learned that conventional stretching could cause real harm, such as muscle pulls and tears. With Jim and Phil's program, the Michigan Women's track team went from eighth in the conference with 60 percent injuries to first in the conference with nearly 0 percent injuries in just one year.

Finally, AI stretching does what stretching is supposed to do. AI reduces your work load in most sports by removing tightness so you can swing your limbs more freely. It transports oxygen to sore muscles and quickly removes toxins from muscles, so recovery is faster. AI stretching works as a deep massage technique because it activates muscle fibers during stretching.

Even if you're a veteran stretcher, you'll be struck by how specifically you stretch exactly where you need it the most. Jim told me, "Isolated Stretching is just that, isolated. It's critical to stretch one muscle at a time. That's what's wrong with the guy in the gym on the floor, trying to touch his knee with his head. He's trying to stretch his back and his hamstrings at the same time. If you do that, you're literally pitting one muscle group against the other, making you more prone to injury."

I've got my whole family doing AI stretching everyday. Try it whenever you're stuck in a line at the airport or bank. It's a great stress reliever. Good luck and enjoy the book.

BOB ARNOT, M.D.
Author of *Dr. Bob Arnot's Guide to Turning Back the Clock*

Contents

Part III: Stretching for Life

Introduction

Active-Isolated Stretching: A Revolution in Athletic Training

Picture the last time you saw a runner stretching before he trotted over to the track. It's always the same, isn't it? Standing behind his car, he throws his leg up onto the trunk, his knee straight and locked. Then he reaches out toward his toes. Bounce. Hold. Bounce. Hold. Hurt. Hold longer. Using the weight of his torso, grabbing onto his calf and pulling himself lower and lower, his hands get closer to those toes with every bounce.

This has to be a successful stretch. His hamstring, the massive muscle in the back of his thigh, is getting warmed up and ready for the explosive workout just about to begin. Right?

WRONG! When a muscle is stretched with bouncing and pulling, it has a natural tendency to protect itself from this violence, however well-intentioned. It quickly contracts back to the range it considers to be normal. Only a *relaxed* muscle will allow itself to be stretched. And the hamstring is not the relaxing muscle in this standard leg-up-on-the-trunk stretch. The muscle on the *other* side of the thigh, the quadricep, is. What does our runner succeed in doing? Alarming the hamstring to tighten in order to protect itself; relaxing the quadricep for a good stretch that never happens; and getting a nasty heel print on the trunk of his car.

More bad news. Our runner's leg-up-on-the-trunk stretch involves literally hundreds of muscles from his upraised ankle to his back, and from his arms to his neck. All those other muscles are tightening up. Like the hamstring, they are contracting into their protective postures.

And here's the final clincher. After our runner's workout, proper stretching would allow his muscles to increase blood flow and oxygenation, and to flush themselves of waste products such as lactic acid. Stretching with bouncing and pulling tightens up every system the muscle uses to heal itself. Nothing good happens. Not only won't our runner recover quickly, but he is setting himself up for an injury.

Instinct and science tell us that stretching is a necessary component in achieving flexibility. Yet the stretching debate has raged since time began, because, frankly, the benefits of stretching are difficult to quantify and results are inconsistent. And now we know why. We were doing it wrong! In the endless quest to maximize human performance, researchers, coaches, trainers, and therapists of world-class athletes and Olympic champions have finally figured it all out. And, to date, it just might be the best kept secret in the world of sports. It's a revolutionary, yet remarkably simple flexibility system called **Active-Isolated Stretching**.

Here's how it works:

1. Prepare to stretch one isolated muscle at a time.

2. Actively contract the muscle that is *opposite* the isolated muscle. The isolated muscle then will relax in preparation for its stretch.

3. Stretch it gently and quickly—hold the stretch for no more than 2 seconds.

4. Release the stretch before the muscle reacts to being stretched (by going into its protective contraction).

5. Do it again.

6. Go out and win.

(I told you it was remarkably simple.)

A flexible body is more efficient, is more easily trained to strength and endurance, enjoys more range of motion, stays balanced more easily, is less prone to injury, recovers from workouts more quickly, and feels better.

As internationally known personal trainers and therapists, we have been using our Active-Isolated Stretching method for years with professional, amateur, and Olympic athletes. But we cannot always travel with our clients or work with them every day, so it has always been important to give them stretching "prescriptions" to take on the road. Through this book, we now share those prescriptions with you.

ACTIVE-ISOLATED STRETCHING: YOUR SECRET TRAINING WEAPON

Let us give you an example of the results of integrating Active-Isolated Stretching into a training program. In evaluating two runners competing in the 1992 New York City Marathon, researchers analyzed their gait patterns and counted their steps. They discovered that, although the gaits of the two were very similar, the runner with the longer stride took fewer steps to cover the 26.2-mile course, ran more comfortably, finished sooner, and recovered more quickly. We have confirmed time and time again that, by increasing flexibility and lengthening stride, a runner can dramatically improve completion time. We are seeing athletes enhance their performance *without* increasing their mileage, spending more time on the track, losing more weight, or taking drugs. When one simple link—Active-Isolated Stretching—is added to the chain, the whole chain gets stronger.

THE 21-DAY GUARANTEE

We don't want to change your fundamental training. All we want to do is add one small component: Active-Isolated Stretching. We want you to make a 21-day commitment to put Active-Isolated Stretching into your training. It takes 21 days for a habit to become ingrained in personal patterns. At the end of your 21-day trial, you will have made such dramatic improvements in your performance that you will never turn back. Active-Isolated Stretching will be part of your training and part of your life.

WHAT BEING AN ATHLETE MEANS

The dictionary defines an athlete as "one who participates in sports or exercise." With a definition as broad as that, almost everyone is an athlete in some way and to some degree. We couldn't agree more. If you make your living at sports, you are a "Professional Athlete." If you participate in sports in your spare time without being paid, you are an "Amateur Athlete." And if you use your body at work, then you are an "Occupational Athlete." No matter which category you're in, you deserve to live, work, play, and love in a body that is performing at its maximum potential. If you are working toward that goal, you are an "Athlete in Training."

You should be in good general health before you begin this or any fitness program. If you are in doubt, please consult your personal physician.

PUTTING ALL THE FITNESS PIECES IN PLACE

This introductory section is our consult with you. Our in-person clients always have questions during their first visits. We've culled the questions asked most often, and we've answered them by identifying twelve myths of exercise approaches and results. Don't skip over the myths; you may be harming yourself by doing something you've always thought was OK.

A good consult is a dialogue, not a monologue. Your participation has two elements:

1. Your commitment to a 21-day trial, which means you'll stick to Active-Isolated Stretching because you've decided to gain its benefits for yourself; "I'll try it if you will" doesn't work, and no group activity is on the agenda.

2. With the guidance we give here, you'll do an honest and sensible evaluation of exactly where you are on day 1 of the 21-day trial. Don't make yourself any more or less fit than you are, because you'll only be counterfeiting your own results. Knowing what your body zones are and what condition each zone is in puts you on the launching pad for the rest of the book.

Self-evaluation is an important step in starting any training program. Your goal is to determine your Flexibility Ranges of Motion—how far you can stretch or flex each muscle group. Once you know those ranges, you'll know where you need to focus your efforts.

In Part I, we present the *Active-Isolated Stretch Catalog*—fifty-nine stretches that involve all the regions (we call them *zones*) of the body. The catalog explains in detail how to perform each stretch, either alone or with the assistance of a partner. The catalog is the "showcase" of the book. You'll refer to it over and over when you put together a stretch routine for a new sport or activity—or for a new season, when you have to restart your moves and skills.

In Part II, we discuss dozens of sports and athletic activities. Each unit begins with a listing of the body zones that will be affected by the activity and should therefore have a high degree of flexibility. For each zone, we give you the numbers of stretches described in Part I that you should concentrate on. Following this customized advice on the stretches you need, a "Coaches' Notes" section covers the challenges, studies and their results, and anatomy "sound bites" specific to the activity. These are the same tips we give our in-person clientele.

Part II connects to a feature that appears at the back of the book: a *Personal Active-Isolated Stretching Program* (pages 231–235). A sample page from the Program appears on the next page here. Your personal notation system depends on which sports—or how many sports, in different seasons—you engage in. If you're a year-round golfer and swimmer, your research on stretches is fairly simple. If your sports choices change drastically with the seasons, or you're centering on a particular event like a marathon, you can adapt our Personal Active-Isolated Stretching Program to your changing stretching needs. Photocopy the pages, make notations that make sense to you, and tape the pages where they're visible in your exercise area. *Voilà!* You've just constructed your own stretching training program.

Part III is directed toward showing expectant moms and older persons the benefits stretching can add to their lives. We'll also discuss ten medical conditions for which proper stretching—not surgery—may be the best cure.

Our message, to all of our readers, is that stretching is relevant throughout your life.

Before we deal with questions and myths about exercise, let's walk through how you should prepare your Personal Active-Isolated Stretching Program sheets. For purposes of our example, let's say that

PERSONAL ACTIVE-ISOLATED STRETCHING PROGRAM

ZONE 1
Upper Legs, Hips and Trunk
(The Foundation)

	NOTES

1. Single Leg Pelvic Tilt
2. Double Leg Pelvic Tilt
3. Bent Leg Hamstrings
4. Straight Leg Hamstrings
5. Hip Adductors
6. Hip Abductors
7. Psoas
8. Quadriceps
9. Gluteals
10. Trunk Rotators
11. Piriformis
12. Hip External Rotators
13. Hip Internal Rotators
14. Medial Hip Rotators
15. Trunk Extensors
16. Thoracic-Lumbar Rotators
17. Lateral Trunk Flexors

Date _____

you're a typist and keyboarder on workdays and a wind surfer whenever the weather and your free time allow.

Begin by looking up your workday athletic activity, titled "Keyboarding All Day," in the Contents. Mark the page and then find the section on "Wind Surfing." Have a set of your personal program sheets ready, and log in the numbers of the specific Active-Isolated Stretches assigned to your occupational activity. Flip to "Wind Surfing," which has also been assigned specific Active-Isolated Stretches. Log those numbers on your sheets. Note that some of the stretches are identical to the ones assigned for your keyboarding activity. One of the surprises in studying the flexibility of the human body is how often you will find an overlap in the use of the joints and muscles. Who would have imagined that some of the same muscles you use to type your name are essential for propelling your Wind Surfer over the crashing waves at 40 miles per hour? And yet it's true.

Next, read carefully the "Coaches' Notes." On keyboarding, they cover such topics as posture, taking breaks, and carpal tunnel syndrome. Turn to "Wind Surfing" and read about body positioning, the anatomical challenges of pulling and rapidly changing position, and the effects of sun and salt water on athletes.

One of the things you will learn as you study sports activities is that the body is like a remarkable computer with all the systems mysteriously and undeniably linked. A flat foot may be the cause of a searing pain in your lower back. A clenched fist may be the cause of a massive cramp between your shoulder blades. And a relaxed and flexible body may help you become a more successful athlete than you ever imagined was possible.

TWELVE MYTHS

In our consult sessions, we've been amazed at some of the myths that have come to light in our clients' questions. We know how this happens. A newcomer to sport, or to workouts in general, wants quick advice on the best route to the inside track. So, in lieu of professional coaching, athletes will default to what we call "Aboriginal Coaching"—information and advice shared by the campfire, one warrior to another. Many athletes will tell you that what they know about their sports was imparted mostly by other athletes. There is nothing wrong with this *as long as the information is accurate*. The problem is that some of the "conventional wisdom" that governs athletes' decisions is WRONG! Even worse, the misinformation has been around so long that it has gained some credibility. You've probably heard the old campfire line: "What you don't know can't hurt you." We disagree. It can. We call the worst pieces of this misinformation "The Twelve Myths." And we want to set the record straight.

Myth 1.   Muscles recover more quickly if I sit in a tub of hot water, right?

WRONG!   Although we will not deny that it feels wonderful to sink into a hot bath after a hard workout, especially on a cold winter's day, we have to tell you that "feeling wonderful" is about the limit of the benefit. External heat is comforting and relaxing, but to facilitate muscle recovery, you need a little more. When your muscles have been active, they already have been heated up. Cold reduces swelling and initially restricts blood flow, providing a natural compress on the microscopic tears in the tissue that are leaking blood into the traumatized area. Shortly, the body will recruit new blood to the cold area (notice it turns a little red?). The new blood flushes out metabolic wastes and lactic acid—byproducts of heavy muscle activity.

If you have a localized "sore spot," you can treat it with a home-made ice pack. We recommend that you fill a paper cup with water and keep it in the freezer. When you need an ice pack, simply peel down the rim to expose the surface of the ice. The paper cup, or what's left of it, serves as a little holder to keep your fingers warm and dry. Gently rub or swirl the ice surface on your injured or traumatized body part. Keep it moving and apply as much pressure as you can stand. For the first minute, it will feel uncomfortable, but this will ease. Treat yourself for five to ten minutes. Watch your skin to make certain that it doesn't turn white, signaling frostbite. If the area you are treating is a little larger, a bag of frozen peas is a wonderfully pliable ice pack that can be refrozen frequently and reused for a long time. For a full-scale treatment (such as for post-marathon soreness), fill a bathtub with cold water and add five to ten bags of ice. Then sink your entire body into the water (the screaming and cursing will subside within a few minutes, and your body will give you an expression of gratitude the next morning).

By the way, do not rely on topical creams and ointments to help you either to "warm up" before a workout or to recover after one. They feel warm and tingly, but they are not going to help a muscle at either end of your workout. If anything, they will give you the delusion that you have done something good for yourself and will delay action that could actually be more helpful.

Myth 2. If I am constantly getting injured on one side, that must mean that I have a leg-length discrepancy, right?

WRONG!   We hear this one all the time, and we are glad to set the record straight! Significant leg-length discrepancies are not that common. Frequently, an athlete who is lying flat on a table, will be evaluated by an observer standing at the foot of the table. The observer takes the athlete's feet in his or her hands, presses the ankles together, "eyeballs" the soles of the feet, and finally declares, "Yep! Your left ankle bone is a full half-inch below your right one, pal! Your left leg definitely is longer." Then the athlete goes out and gets a half-inch lift for the right shoe so that both legs can be even. This apparent leg-length discrepancy probably is caused NOT by a leg bone that is longer, but by an imbalance in the muscles and tendons of the pelvis, the foundation of the body. And the source of this imbalance might surprise you. A tight hamstring on one side can jack the other side of the pelvis up. A tight iliotibial band on one side could jack the other side of the pelvis up. The imbalance is common in people who do one thing in the same way all the time, such as a runner who sprints around a track in one direction day after day. Tennis players who develop their *upper* bodies on one side because they swing their rackets with their dominant hands can experience imbalance in the muscles that affect the pelvis. When the pelvic region—hips and trunk—is free-floating and flexible, an apparent leg-length discrepancy may "mysteriously" disappear.

Myth 3. Resting or immobilizing an exhausted or injured muscle will facilitate healing, right?

WRONG!   Conventional wisdom used to be: RICE an injury. Treat it with *R*est, *I*ce, *C*ompression, and *E*levation. But, we have found that immobilizing an injury—unless a fracture or a shredded muscle is involved—shuts the muscle down and restricts blood flow. Opening up a muscle or joint, and encouraging blood flow to oxygenate the area and flush out metabolic waste from the injury, seems a whole lot more intelligent. Additionally, immobilizing a muscle causes it—and everything around it—to atrophy. The body instantly will launch a series of compensations to make up for the fact that something is not working properly (or at all), which will cause more imbalances and instabilities and greater risk of more injury.

Tom Nohilly, the 1989 NCAA Champion in 3,000-meter steeple-chase, was competing well in the 1992 Olympic Trials in New Orleans . . . until the semifinal heat. In the kind of sickening moment that every athlete dreads, Tom hit a barrier at top speed. When he crumpled to the track, his ankle was on fire. Following exact injury protocol for an Olympic Trial, experienced athletic trainers took him off the track, diagnosed a sprain, taped him to constrict the swelling, and expressed their heartfelt sympathy at his obvious inability to compete in the finals, which were just two days away. Tom was devastated. Because we were working in the infield and are good friends with Tom, we offered our assistance and took him to our stretch table. His ankle was black and blue, and swollen to the size of a grapefruit. We untaped it and iced him immediately. Working slowly and very gently to restore a tiny range of motion, we "pumped" his ankle to get blood to the area. Within an hour of ice application and Active-Isolated Stretching, the swelling was diminished sufficiently for him to walk (gingerly). For two days, we worked continuously on icing and stretching. Two days after he was carried from the track, he placed fourth in the Olympic Trials, barely missing a U.S. Olympic Team berth.

So here's our opinion on the best treatment: *MICE* an injury. *M*ove it, *I*ce it, *C*ompress it when you're on periodic breaks from your rehab program, and *E*levate it (preferably with your stretch rope, during long and frequent routines). Now that we've spelled that out, let us add that you must be VERY certain that you're not dealing with a catastrophic injury such as a fracture. Get a good diagnosis from a physician if you're in doubt. And move carefully and gently. Even the tiniest range of motion is extremely helpful.

Myth 4. I must always warm up before I stretch, right?

WRONG! Stretching IS warming up. As you work your muscles, you are pumping blood to them and firing them, one at a time. As each set of stretches progresses, you gradually increase your range of motion with gentle assistance at the end of each stretch. Each subsequent stretch is a little more elongated, which means the muscle on top of the stretching muscle is firing a little harder. Everything is becoming more efficient and working more smoothly. This is why we recommend an Active-Isolated Stretch routine before you begin a workout.

Following a workout, an identical routine can help flush metabolic wastes such as lactic acid, which accumulate in a stressed muscle. The gentle pumping action of the routine sends blood to parts of the body that have worked hard. Healing and recovery begin and are accelerated. Range of motion is restored in areas that have been tracked in very rigid and specific patterns—during running, for example. For these reasons, stretching is recommended as a "cool-down" routine.

Myth 5. I should hold a stretch from ten seconds to three minutes in order for it to do me any good, right?

WRONG! Muscles can elongate, when they're healthy, up to 1.6 times their length, but they generally don't react well to that much stretching. If you elongate a muscle too quickly or too far, it automatically and ballistically recoils to protect itself from ripping. This compensation, called a "myotatic reflex," kicks in at *three seconds*. Imagine yourself the last time you tried to do splits. Unless you are unusually flexible, the sequence went something like this. You leapt out of the chair and stood straight up on the floor. You slid your right foot forward and your left foot backward until you felt a "tug" on the insides of your thighs. You either pulled up immediately or buckled your knees and dropped to the floor to get that pressure off your hips. You drew your knees up to relax the tension. You were experiencing the myotatic reflex: a loud and clear message to you that you were going rip within the next second, and you needed to let go NOW.

The trick in progressing in flexibility is to stretch a muscle, but not allow it time to engage the myotatic reflex. You work quickly and gently. The muscle you are stretching is totally relaxed because the muscle on top of it is doing all the work. The stretching muscle never has time to fire. Because it is stretched, held for two seconds, and released, it doesn't need to protect itself. The myotatic reflex is never engaged.

Myth 6. Drink when I'm thirsty, right?

WRONG! If you wait until you feel thirsty and then start to drink, it's too late. Thirst is a symptom of dehydration, and dehydration decreases blood volume. With less blood getting to the skin, the systems that control heat dissipation fail. Once this happens, an athlete overheats even more quickly. Performance levels drop, and things can get dangerous. Symptoms of dehydration include muscle cramping, excessive sweating, dark urine or infrequent urination, weakness, nausea, rapid heart rate, headache, light-headedness, increased body core temperature, heat exhaustion, and heat stroke. In extreme cases, the consequences of dehydration can be fatal. It makes no difference whether you are working out in cold or hot weather, inside or outside, in arid or humid climates, on a ski slope or in a swimming pool—hydration is vitally important.

You should plan to hydrate before, during, and after your workout. Plain (filtered) water is good, but some athletes prefer "sports drinks"— beverages that hydrate, replace electrolytes lost in sweating, and contain carbohydrates such as glucose, sucrose, fructose, and glucose polymers. Some experts believe it is best to drink water before your workout for hydration, and turn to sports drinks later during your workout, when your body needs the carbohydrates and is prepared to handle and use the sugars you're taking in. There are a lot of good sports drinks on the market. Because results and reactions vary with individuals, you need to test them during training. Our consulting dietitian, Kathryn A. Parker, R.D., L.D., tells us that, no matter what you drink, it will absorb more quickly if you drink it cold (40° is optimum) and more slowly if it has a high sugar content.

Myth 7. If muscles are flexible around a joint, I could get injured. I should be tight to perform better, right?

WRONG! It's easy to see where this attitude comes from. Even we have said to an injured athlete, "You have weak knees. You need to get stronger." It is logical to assume that if you build a tight, bulky musculature, you can protect a joint, but protection is not that simple. There is a BIG difference between a strong muscle and a tight one. A tight muscle can be very weak and offer virtually no protection for a joint. A tight muscle is an inefficient muscle. It cannot elongate and then reflex quickly to make a joint move. It takes too much energy to move it. It doesn't fire quickly on command, and you have to recruit extra muscles to assist it. It's prone to injury because you can't move it fast enough or position yourself well enough to avoid trauma or effects of overuse. It tracks rigidly and has a limited range of movement. And when a movable force meets an immovable object, something's got to give—whether or not it should.

Power is the combination of strength and flexibility. Tightness doesn't help—in fact, it hurts.

Myth 8. Injuries are inevitable, right?

WRONG! Dave Martin, an Olympic Coach and the U.S. Track and Field Cross-Country National Championships in San Francisco in

1989, once wisely noted, "Injury is a mistake in your training program." Well-trained athletes should never get hurt (unless there's a collision or similar accident). Injury is entirely avoidable if you properly apply knowledge and basic principles. We urge our athletes to take charge, to train and compete with intelligence, and to be always in pursuit of better nutrition, better rest, and better training methods. Injuries rarely "just happen." Sadly, when we look back over events that led to an injury, we can find clear indicators that it was forthcoming— and there are usually several of these indicators. We coach our athletes to pay attention to subtle and not-so-subtle "warning signs": tightness, soreness, recovery that seems sluggish, cramping, sharp little pains, aching, fatigue, sleeplessness, changes in attitude, feeling "off," and so on. Warning signs vary with each circumstance, so we encourage a daily "inventory." Suspicious symptoms are evaluated immediately and completely, and adjustments are made to prevent injury.

Wise athletes remember that training and competing aren't the only possible ways to sustain an injury. Life can be a contact sport, and an injury totally unrelated to your sport can shut you down.

Myth 9.   The older I get, the less flexible I'll become, right?

WRONG!   As you grow older, there is no need to grunt and groan when you get out of a chair, or shuffle when you walk or turn your whole body to look at what's beside you. Experts acknowledge a biological decrease in natural flexibility as a person ages, but there is growing evidence that the decreases in physical function we commonly associate with aging are not entirely related to advancing years, but are attributable, in large part, to a sedentary lifestyle. When aging is accompanied by an increasingly sedentary lifestyle, muscle atrophy is almost always the result. And once that happens, it is difficult to regain the earlier muscle mass with strength training and to regain the former flexibility with stretching, although it can be done.

There are compelling reasons to avoid a sedentary lifestyle. Improved nutrition and medical discoveries have made it possible for us to live longer, so taking care of these bodies in which we are going to live for a long time is increasingly important. Researchers tell us that a decline in flexibility means a decline in stability, balance, and mobility, which contributes to the falls that can be deadly to the elderly. Equally deadly is restriction of spinal mobility, which causes compression and severe impediments in cardiovascular function. Following the axiom "Move it or lose it!" may mean saving your life—literally.

Apparently, it is never too late to start with *aerobic, strength,* and *flexibility* training. Researchers have found that programmed, regular exercise (three days a week, twenty to thirty minutes per session) significantly improves all three in both men and women. To prolong life and preserve a good quality of life, working out is important.

Myth 10. **Flat feet and fallen arches are corrected by support devices that are put inside the shoe, right?**

WRONG! Walking and running place impressive demands on the feet, no question about it. But a foot is remarkable in its shock-absorbing abilities. If you are like most of us, as you walk or run, when you put your forward foot down on the surface, your rear foot rolls to the inside. As the full impact of your footstrike spreads throughout your foot, your shin rotates internally, taking your foot with it and converting your foot to a shock absorber. The subtalar joint (on top of your foot, where the ankle joins the foot) converts the vertical force to longitudinal force, spreading the shock through your entire foot. You adjust the torque to the surface on which you're walking or running, and then, continuing in forward motion, you instantaneously rotate your foot to the outside. Your foot then returns to being rigid, which allows you to lift off again. It's a wonderful, miraculous process. The arch of your foot acts like a spring or a shock absorber. It takes the "hit" from your foot plant and keeps it from jarring your knee and hip. If you put a support in your shoe, you are guaranteeing that your "spring" has nowhere to go and your shock absorber can't absorb shock. It will feel good temporarily, because it will relieve tension in your foot and leg, but, long-term, it will accomplish nothing. In fact, it will fool you and keep you from looking for a solution to your problem.

It's far more intelligent to try to strengthen your arch so that it will work properly. We recommend four to six weeks of progressive strength training along with your Active-Isolated Stretching program. Stand on a phone book with your feet forward, your toes and the balls of your feet on the book, and your heels suspended over the edge. Brace yourself so you won't slip. Maintaining complete control, stand up on your toes and then slowly lower your heels toward the floor until you feel a gentle pull. Return to the tip-toe position and repeat ten times. Turn your toes toward each other—pigeon-toed style—and repeat the exercise. Turn your toes outward and repeat the exercise.

For your next strengthening exercise, you will need a chair or other hard surface; a long, tube-style sock; and a one-pound can of beans (or equivalent). Put the can of beans in the toe of the sock. Take your shoes off. Sit on the edge of a sturdy chair and lift one knee until your bare foot is tucked up on the seat, with your heel against your buttock. Take the sock with the can in the toe and wrap or tie it around your foot so that the weight of the can dangles between your big toe and the toe next to it. Hang the ball of your foot and your toes straight out over the edge of the chair, keeping your heel on the seat. Grip the sock (and can) with your toes and lift ten times. Rest. Lift again ten times. Switch feet and repeat. Gradually, as you get stronger, use heavier cans until you can lift a five-pound can.

Finally, take the can out of the sock and put it on the far end of a towel you have laid on the floor. Sit at the opposite end of the towel and put your bare foot at the edge. Grip the towel in your toes and bunch it up, pulling the can toward you. Keep gripping and bunching until you have moved the can all the way. Straighten up the towel, replace the can, switch feet, and repeat the maneuver. Remember, as you increase the weight of the can in your sock-lift, use the same heavier can in your towel-grip.

To test your progress, get your bare foot wet and step onto the sidewalk, a shower tile, or some other surface where you can leave an imprint. The goal is to have your footprints resemble a "C" (left foot) and its mirror image (right foot). The bigger the open space on the inside of a foot, the higher the arch and the greater your ability to spring or absorb shock.

Myth 11. **Inflammation of the muscle or joint can be healed completely with anti-inflammatory medications and bracing, right?**

WRONG! Aspirin and nonsteroidal anti-inflammatory drugs (NSAIDs) such as ibuprofen do have a purpose. Taken properly, they can reduce pain and inflammation in joints and soft tissues, such as muscles and ligaments, by blocking the production of prostaglandins (chemicals that cause inflammation and trigger transmission of the pain signal to the brain). When you are in pain, you tense up to protect the injury from further harm. Your whole body forms a kind of "splint." Protection takes enormous energy and causes imbalances and tension everywhere. Additionally, you don't sleep well when you are hurting, and whenever your rest is disturbed, your ability to cope with the injury and make good decisions is diminished.

To start the healing process, take advantage of the comfort levels afforded to you by proper dosage of a painkiller. Feeling better may allow you to move an injured joint or flex an injured muscle just a little, so that you have less need to protect yourself. You'll be more relaxed. You'll sleep better, allowing your body to rejuvenate more quickly. And, most important, when you feel comfortable, you will be able to move, increase your range of motion, and pump blood to the injury to promote healing.

A few words of caution: Pain is your body's way of communicating clear messages to you about the status of an injury. Don't use painkillers to mask pain that you need to be evaluating and using for information on treatment. We had one client who took ibuprofen, masked the pain of a stress fracture in her shin, and continued to run—with disastrous long-term consequences. Also, keep in mind that even a product bought "over the counter" is still a medication. NSAIDs have possible side effects of which you need to be aware: nausea, indigestion, diarrhea, and peptic ulcers. Aspirin could cause clotting disorders, prolonged bleeding, colitis, gastrointestinal disorders, ringing in the ears, and aggravation of asthma, hives, and gout. Be careful.

Myth 12. Improvement of sports performance comes from working harder. To progress, I need to be out there every day, hammering as hard as I can, right?

WRONG! You need to rest. The sports performance cycle works like this: In a workout, you stress a muscle or a system, literally tearing it down. The muscle or system remodels or rebuilds, coming back a little stronger. You stress it again and tear it down. It rebuilds even more strongly. You stress it again and tear it down. It rebuilds, getting stronger every time. If the interval between workouts (the tearing-down phases of the cycle) is insufficient, you do not give your body time to rebuild. You change the cycle from "tearing down/building up/tearing down/building up" to "tearing down/tearing down/tearing down/tearing down." It doesn't take long for the cycle to fail. The key to successful progression in getting stronger is to honor the interval of time needed for your body to rebuild—roughly 48 hours. This doesn't mean that you can be active only every other day. It just means that you must do different things or do things at different intensities on sequential days. The rest day in between "hammerings" will allow the rebuilding, and you'll get full benefit from your workout.

How do you know if you're overtraining? Good clues are: rapid pulse before you get out of bed in the morning, soreness, tightness, unexplained colds, sleep disorders, crankiness, and lack of progress.

Or an honest look at your training log that reveals hard training seven days a week.

YOUR PERSONAL DECISION AND COMMITMENT

Let's review what we've covered so far in this initial consult section.

- The list of sports and occupational activities we'll be discussing in detail.

- The basics of how Active-Isolated Stretching works.

- The 21-day commitment to put Active-Isolated Stretching into your training routine.

- The need to do an honest evaluation of your fitness level.

- The Personal Active-Isolated Stretching Program format and how to use it.

- A dozen myths about training methods—and the reasons to change your thinking.

Beginning with the next section on ranges of flexibility, your involvement in Active-Isolated Stretching gets under way. Through this book, we take you on as a "client." We *know* the benefits of Active-Isolated Stretching, and we're ready to pass them along to you. But the signpost at this point reads: YOU HAVE TO STRETCH.

It's important to understand that there is no magic in our method. Active-Isolated Stretching offers you a unique tool, but it is up to you to use it. You'll learn its benefits as you earn them during your 21-day trial. Why have we asked you to commit for only 21 days? Because we know that:

- Stretching will become a habit in that amount of time.

- Anyone can do anything for three short weeks.

- At the end of that time, your athletic performance will be so improved, and you will feel so good, that you won't be tempted to quit.

Getting started is the hardest part, trust us. Here's how to do it in three steps:

1. Make a decision to put Active-Isolated Stretching into your workout. Make that decision *once*. Do not remake it again and again. For example, decide that you are going to get up 20 minutes earlier every morning so that you can integrate a stretching routine into your workout. Decide that *once*. Do not even consider renegotiating it every morning. The alarm goes off, and you get up. No discussion. Within minutes, you begin your stretching.

2. Make a commitment. You've promised yourself something good. Follow through.

3. Do it. Show up on time, know the routine, get down on the floor and do it. Simple.

The rewards of Active-Isolated Stretching will far outweigh the inconveniences of integrating a short new routine into your workout. This book is a step-by-step guide to the techniques and tools that have been developed over many years in sports clinics, venues, and training camps all over the world. Together, we will help you reach your maximum performance potential.

HOW FLEXIBLE ARE YOU?

We've referred to the need to do an honest evaluation of your fitness level. Here is the method that we believe gives the best reading.

When we begin to work with an athlete, the first thing we do is evaluate his or her Flexibility Range. Back in the Dark Ages of training, we used the "Sit and Reach Test." An athlete would sit on the floor with his or her back up against the wall and a yardstick placed on the floor between his or her knees, parallel to his or her legs. The athlete would reach toward his or her toes, and the point where his or her fingertips touched the yardstick indicated the degree of the athlete's flexibility. The problem was that this stretch involved many muscles and there was no way to tell which specific muscle was flexible. We now know that the short reach that used to be proclaimed the sign of a "tight lower back" might well have been a loose lower back with tight hamstrings.

Our Active-Isolated Stretching method gives you a much more accurate tool. You will be measuring 59 muscles and muscle groups that affect your joints' range of motion. Our method divides the body into five zones:

Zone 1	Upper Legs, Hips, and Trunk (The Foundation)
Zone 2	Shoulders
Zone 3	Neck
Zone 4	Arms, Elbows, Wrists, and Hands
Zone 5	Lower Legs, Ankles, and Feet

Some of the flexibility ranges are subdivided into left side and right side. Balance—similar ranges on both sides—is important to maximize athletic performance and prevent injury.

Each muscle in each zone has its own Flexibility Range of Motion. For these ranges, we use a double labeling system—the name of a color and a word description. Here's a quick key to the double labels and their meaning:

Red Range:	This muscle is too tight. It is going to cause problems.
Yellow Range:	This muscle is in the normal range. Not bad. Not good.
Green Range:	This is an elite athlete's muscle. Here is where you want to be.
Blue Range:	This muscle is hypermobile—going beyond the range. No problem, but you need to make certain that you are strong enough to compensate.

Memorize these labels and their meanings so that they're as familiar as your first name. Your Flexibility Range of Motion is stated in numbers, and the key will be your frame of reference.

Your goal should be to get yourself into the GREEN RANGE as far as possible. In other words, if you are in the GREEN RANGE, congratulations; but keep working on your Flexibility Range of Motion until your numbers are well up within that range. The greater the number of degrees a muscle moves, the better.

YOU'LL LEARN THE RIGHT WAY TO STRETCH

As you evaluate each Flexibility Range of Motion, you'll be learning how to do the stretching, and you'll be studying the basic anatomy involved. Remember that this is ACTIVE-ISOLATED Stretching. We'll tell you which muscles you need to activate—or to *contract*—and which muscles you need to isolate and stretch. Some stretches are very simple. Some are more complicated and require the use of a rope or belt looped around a body part to help you get a little "tug" at the end of a stretch. If you enjoy working with a training partner, we'll show you how an assistant can help you get the most out of a stretch.

Can a Muscle Stretch or Flex Too Far?

Not without a lot of pain. You can stretch a muscle 1.6 times its length, but Mother Nature designed human anatomy to limit ranges of motion and prevent injury. How flexible you can become is to a certain extent influenced by genetics. You are limited by your bone conformations, and frankly, some people are built to flex more than others. You won't always be able to get to the GREEN RANGE, but perseverance will bring you to the maximum of your own flexibility.

A muscle *can* be stretched to the point of ripping in an accident; fortunately, accidents are uncommon in training.

Can I Be Too Flexible?

No, but like a ballet dancer or a hurdler, you must accompany high GREEN RANGE or BLUE RANGE flexibility with strength and balance.

CONDUCTING YOUR OWN FLEXIBILITY EVALUATION

To evaluate your body just as we would, find a two-hour block of uninterrupted time and invest it in your training program.

Dress in loose-fitting clothing, move back the furniture if necessary, and assemble the following:

- An eight-foot rope, or two fabric belts tied together securely.
- A set of Range of Motion Evaluation worksheets (photocopy pages 236–240).
- A pen or pencil, to record your measurements (you can use red, yellow, green, and blue markers if you want to get fancy).
- A clock with a large face, or a clock face, numbered correctly from 1 to 12, drawn on a paper plate.
- A large mirror, positioned so that you can see yourself when you're standing or lying down.

Each of your joints has a specific, measurable Flexibility Range of Motion. We give you three ways to measure:

1. A statement of the actual degrees of movement
2. A clock face, as a way of visualizing how the positions of the numbers link to angles of your joints
3. A color coding system that puts each Range of Motion into a sort of traffic light context—"red" means muscles are stopped, "yellow" means caution, "green" means all system are GO!, and "blue" means your range is off the chart.

In Part I, you will begin to methodically work your way through the 59 stretches assigned to the body's five zones. You will isolate the muscle or muscle group you are evaluating, contract the opposite muscle, and stretch each isolated muscle or muscle group until it resists slightly.

Next, using a clock face (a real one, or your paper-plate version) as a sort of homemade protractor, you will measure how many degrees your joints move as your muscles stretch and flex. Where we can, our diagrams will show you where to position the center of the clock face as you stretch. If you are unable to "feel" your position, check your position in the large mirror that you have propped up on the floor. For example, lie on your back, lock your right knee, and lift your right leg straight up from the hip. Position the clock face at your hip so that the perpendicular position of your leg aligns with high noon on the clock.

Your position is then at 90° and in the YELLOW RANGE (normal). If you can get your leg to 2:00 or 110°, then you are in the GREEN RANGE (elite athlete) and doing much better.

You will notice that some of the stretches terminate before they enter a BLUE RANGE. This means that the end of the stretch is blocked by your body or the floor.

In most stretches, you will readily feel your position or will be able to check it in the mirror. For example, when you're standing and you lift your arm, it's easy enough to tell whether you can lift it to 9:00, 11:00, or high noon. When you're lying on your back, it may not be easy to check your mirror for an accurate reading on your position. In those situations—or simply to keep yourself "honest"—you might want to enlist the help of a friend (or partner or spouse) to keep the measurements. In fact, the buddy system can contribute to the success of an exercise program. Alternating in the stretching and the assisting roles, you and a friend can measure each other's flexibility and later work out as a pair.

Once you know your present flexibility range, you'll know which muscles need the most work to get into the GREEN RANGE. At the end of three weeks, monitor your progress. Then check yourself again every weeks. How quickly you progress toward the GREEN RANGE, or whether you reach it at all, will depend on a lot of factors. We can't guarantee that you'll "get the green" every time, but, using Active-Isolated Stretching, you *will* improve your flexibility and gain the benefits that the improvement brings.

Now let's get started measuring your flexibility, zone by zone.

Part I

The Active-Isolated Stretch Catalog

*T*his is it! Your commitment has brought you to the stretches that will give you the edge in your sports moves and your everyday activities.

You've promised yourself that you are going to stick to this program for at least 21 days. (We aren't going to worry your 22nd day. You'll be so amazed at the improvements in your sports performance, and at how good you feel, that you'll continue of your own accord.)

To get started on your stretches, there are just a few more things to do:

1. Dress in loose-fitting clothing.

2. Find a place to work out where you will be comfortable. (Our top three choices are on your bed, on a massage table, or on a carpeted floor or a floor mat.)

3. Have your eight-foot length of rope or your tied-together belts handy.

4. Tape the photocopied pages of your Personal Active-Isolated Stretching Program (see page xxviii) on a nearby wall or on the floor near you, so that you can make notes easily. (Or, enlist a partner's help.)

5. Get ready for some real fun.

You'll notice that, for each of the 59 stretches, we tell you what you're stretching (the antagonist) and what you're contracting (the agonist). We give you a detailed description and an illustration of each stretch. In many of the stretches, we've included a section titled "When Two Heads Are Better Than One." This offers a modification that includes the assistance of another person. If you can't find an assistant, no problem. Your rope will give you all the help you need. If you're a professional trainer, this section will tell you how to work out with a client. Also note that some of the stretches eliminate help—such as neck stretches (these are safer if they're solo) or hand stretches (unless you *like* to hold hands, there is no need to assist).

Now you're ready.

MAJOR POSTERIOR MUSCLES

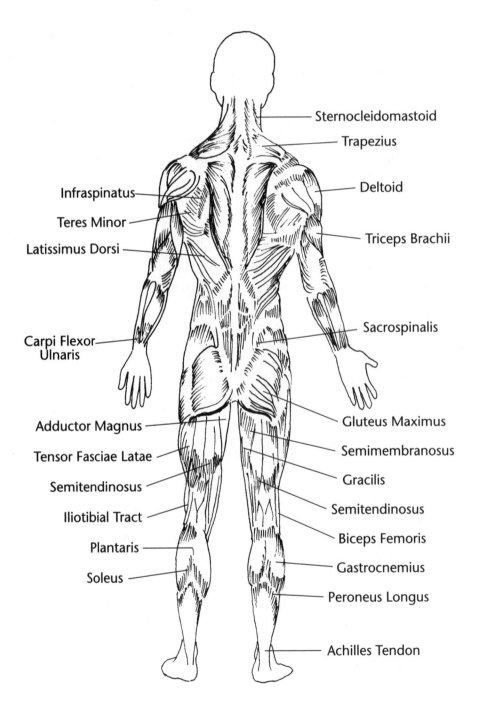

Sternocleidomastoid

Trapezius

Deltoid

Infraspinatus

Teres Minor

Triceps Brachii

Latissimus Dorsi

Sacrospinalis

Carpi Flexor
Ulnaris

Gluteus Maximus

Adductor Magnus

Semimembranosus

Tensor Fasciae Latae

Gracilis

Semitendinosus

Semitendinosus

Iliotibial Tract

Biceps Femoris

Plantaris

Gastrocnemius

Soleus

Peroneus Longus

Achilles Tendon

MAJOR ANTERIOR MUSCLES

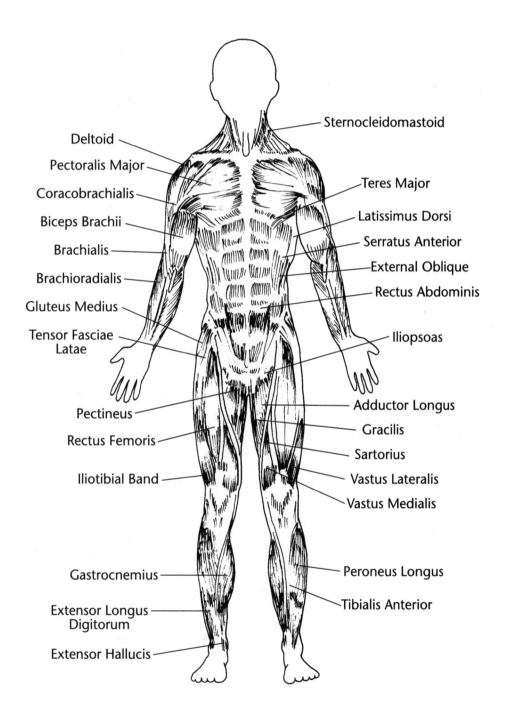

Deltoid

Pectoralis Major

Coracobrachialis

Biceps Brachii

Brachialis

Brachioradialis

Gluteus Medius

Tensor Fasciae Latae

Pectineus

Rectus Femoris

Iliotibial Band

Gastrocnemius

Extensor Longus Digitorum

Extensor Hallucis

Sternocleidomastoid

Teres Major

Latissimus Dorsi

Serratus Anterior

External Oblique

Rectus Abdominis

Iliopsoas

Adductor Longus

Gracilis

Sartorius

Vastus Lateralis

Vastus Medialis

Peroneus Longus

Tibialis Anterior

You might be a little intimidated at first, when you see the number of stretches suggested for each activity ("WHAT? Thirty-nine stretches just to go cross-country skiing?"). But, you'll be holding each stretch for only about 2 seconds, and many require few repetitions, so your entire stretch routine will take only about 20 minutes.

Give yourself a little extra time when you first begin Active-Isolated Stretching. It's bound to take a bit longer when you're learning the exercises. They will quickly become second nature, and you'll soon be moving through your preworkout routine in 15 to 20 minutes. Remember: Give yourself three weeks to fully appreciate the benefits of this new way of stretching. That's how long it will take to fall into a natural Active-Isolated Stretching rhythm and SEE the results.

Keep in mind, too, the incredible muscle structure you are working with. Athletes sometimes take muscular functioning as a "given." You may not remember the anatomical names, but take a good look at the rear (posterior) and front (anterior) views of the intricate system that allows humans to move at all (pages 4 and 5). Care for it as a gift and never take it for granted.

HOW TO STRETCH

Read the instructions for a stretch and picture yourself doing what is described. Identify and isolate the muscle or muscle group you want to stretch. Contract the *opposite* muscle. This will cause the isolated muscle or muscle group to relax automatically. And when it is relaxed, it is ready to stretch. Gently and quickly stretch the isolated muscle. When the muscle has reached the limit of its Range of Motion—that is, when you can stretch it no farther—give yourself a gentle assist. Use your hands, or loop your rope (or belts) around the extremity, and gently pull. How far should the stretch go? Until you experience a slight irritation. We describe it as being a little more than "awareness" and a little less than pain. Stretching should not hurt—ever! Hold the stretch no more than 2 seconds. Remember, when a muscle perceives that it is being forced into a stretch, it contracts to protect itself from being overstretched and ripped. This is called the "myotatic reflex." You want to avoid it. If you can sneak up on a muscle and give it a 2-second stretch without causing it to contract, then you have made progress in extending your Range of Motion.

HOW TO BE A PARTNER

If you are assisting an athlete with stretching, you are there to help, but not too much. Let the athlete do all the work in isolating the muscle to be stretched and firing the opposite muscle. You are there to make sure that proper form is followed, to help set a rhythm, to count, and to assist at the end of each stretch.

Assisting at the end of each stretch is your most important function. When the athlete cannot extend a Range of Motion any farther, you gently extend that range by pressing (or pulling) at the end of the stretch. Hold the stretch for no more than 2 seconds. If you are not particularly strong or if you are smaller than your athlete, there will be a tendency to use your whole body for leverage. If you do, keep your balance so that you do not "fall" into the stretch and accidentally injure your athlete. Keep your fingertips on the muscles being stretched and be sensitive to the "feel" of the muscle. You can tell when it is getting ready to contract because it will quiver or tighten. Additionally, learn to "read" your athlete's face. Look for signs of discomfort, which will indicate that you need to back off immediately.

THE ROUTINES

The 59 routines are assigned to the body's 5 zones. For easy reference, we're repeating them here:

Zone 1	Upper Legs, Hips, and Trunk (The Foundation)
Zone 2	Shoulders
Zone 3	Neck
Zone 4	Arms, Elbows, Wrists, and Hands
Zone 5	Lower Legs, Ankles, and Feet

Each routine works within one zone of the body by unlocking muscles in a specific sequence. Plan to do the routines in order, zone by zone. Very simply, isolate the muscles you want to stretch by contracting the muscles that are *opposite*. The isolated muscles are forced to relax; they can then be stretched. When you have reach the limit of your Range of

Motion—that is, you have gone as far as you can go—use your hands or your rope (or belts) to assist you at the end of the stretch. Stretch until you feel a very slight irritation. Hold for no more than 2 seconds. Release. Return to your original position. Repeat. When done properly, the routine will have a distinct rhythm with no hesitation between stretches.

How Many Times Should I Repeat a Stretch?

Plan to do 10 repetitions of each stretch.

How Long Does Stretching Take?

Ten repetitions of each stretch take under 2 minutes. You'll soon be able to do a solid routine in about 20 minutes. When you first begin, expect to be a little slow as you consult your instructions and fumble with your rope. Be patient. In a short time, you will be rocketing through the stretch routines.

When Should I Stretch?

Stretching right before a workout will warm up your muscles (both the contracted muscles and the stretched muscles) and get them ready for action. Stretching after activity will help relax the muscles and flush out metabolic waste that accumulated during exertion. You will be less sore and will heal more quickly.

If you are not working out or engaging in strenuous activity, we recommend stretching first thing in the morning or right before you go to bed at night. Stretch every day.

What If Time Is Limited?

If your time is limited, you still have some options. Do fewer repetitions of each stretch—but no fewer than 5. Resist the temptation to skip some of the stretches. They are designed in sequences that unlock muscles and joints methodically. Skipping a stretch may lead you into the next stretch in the routine without proper preparation and warm-up. A better time-saving strategy is to limit your workout to a single complete routine. If you can do only one routine, work out in Zone 1, Upper Legs, Hips, and Trunk—the foundation of the body. You'll complete the routine in less than 20 minutes.

Let's Get Started!

Zone 1

Upper Legs, Hips, and Trunk
(The Foundation)

1 Single-Leg Pelvic Tilt

Zone 1

What You Stretch:	Lower back (sacrospinalis) and buttocks (gluteus maximus)
What You Contract:	Abdominals and muscles from the front of the hips down the front of the thighs (hip flexors—including the quadriceps)
How Many Repetitions:	10 each side
How Long to Hold:	2 seconds

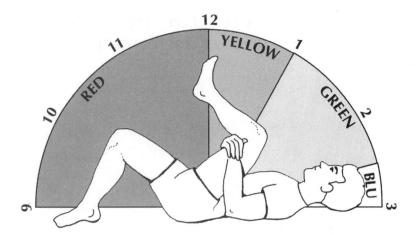

Lie on your back. Bend your nonexercising knee so that you release pressure on your back. Flex (bend) your exercising knee and place your hands behind your knee/thigh to prevent pressure on your knee and provide a little assistance toward the end of the free movement. Using your abdominals and hip flexors, lift your exercising leg toward your chest until you can go no farther. Aim your knee toward your armpit. Gently assist your leg at the end of the stretch with your hands, but do not pull.

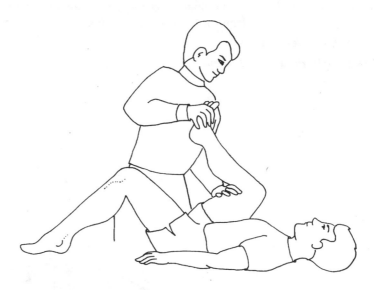

Assistant, let your athlete do all the work, but provide gentle assistance at the end. Place one hand on the back of the thigh and one hand on the heel. Apply a little push for a 2-second hold.

Range	Position on Clock	Degree of Range of Motion
Red Range Too tight	9:00–12:00	0°–90°
Yellow Range Normal	12:00–1:00	90°–120°
Green Range Elite athlete	1:00–2:30	120°–165°
Blue Range Hypermobile	2:30–3:00	165°–180°

2 Double-Leg Pelvic Tilt

What You Stretch:	Lower back (sacrospinalis) and buttocks (gluteus maximus)
What You Contract:	Abdominals and muscles from the front of the hips down the front of the thighs (hip flexors—including the quadriceps)
How Many Repetitions:	10
How Long to Hold:	2 seconds

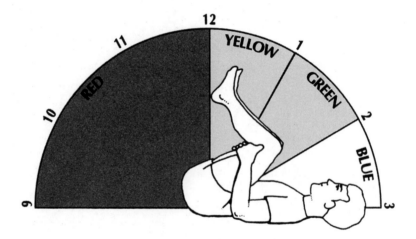

Lie on your back. Begin with both knees bent and your feet flat on the surface on which you are lying. Place your hands behind your knees/thighs to prevent pressure on the knees and provide a little assistance toward the end of the free movement. Using your abdominals and quadriceps, lift your legs toward your chest until you can go no farther. Gently assist with your hands, but do not pull.

When Two Heads Are Better Than One . . .

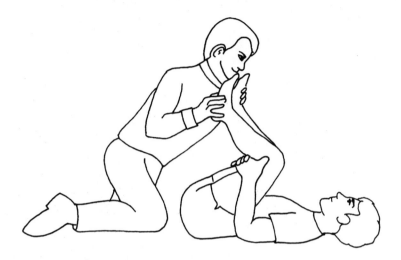

Assistant, place yourself at your athlete's feet. Let your athlete do all the work, but provide gentle assistance at the end. Apply a little push for a 2-second hold.

Range	Position on Clock	Degree of Range of Motion
Red Range Too tight	9:00–12:00	0°–90°
Yellow Range Normal	12:00–1:00	90°–120°
Green Range Elite athlete	1:00–2:00	120°–150°
Blue Range Hypermobile	2:00–3:00	150°–180°

3 Bent-Leg Hamstrings

What You Stretch:	Large muscles in the back of the thighs, just behind the knees (hamstring distal attachments)
What You Contract:	Front of the thighs (quadriceps)
How Many Repetitions:	10 each side
How Long to Hold:	2 seconds

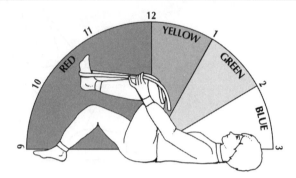

Lie on your back. Begin with both knees bent and your feet flat on the surface on which you are lying. Take your rope and hold the ends together so that it forms a loop. Place the foot of the leg you're exercising into the loop. Lift your leg until your thigh is perpendicular to the surface (your knee is at high noon).

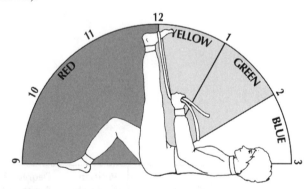

Grasp the ends of the rope (to maintain the loop) with one hand. Place the other hand on top of the thigh of the exercising leg to stabilize it. Gradually extend your leg by contracting your quadriceps. This will cause your foot to rise toward the ceiling. The goal is to lock your knee and have your foot at high noon. You may have to lower the angle of your leg from the hip at first. Use the rope for gentle assistance at the end of the stretch. Do not pull the leg into position or you will irritate the back of your knee.

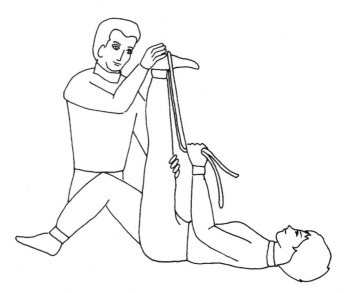

Assistant, help your athlete keep the thigh stable. Let your athlete do all the work and use the rope, but provide gentle assistance at the end. Place one hand on the top of the thigh and one hand on the heel. Apply a little push for a 2-second hold. As the joint opens up, each successive stretch could be a little deeper, bringing the upper thigh closer to the body.

Range	Position on Clock	Degree of Range of Motion
Red Range Too tight	9:00–12:00	0°–90°
Yellow Range Normal	12:00–1:00	90°–120°
Green Range Elite athlete	1:00–2:00	120°–150°
Blue Range Hypermobile	2:00–3:00	150°–180°

4 Straight-Leg Hamstrings

What You Stretch: Large muscles in the back of the thighs (the hamstrings)

What You Contract: Muscles from the front of the hips down the front of the thighs (hip flexors—including the quadriceps)

How Many Repetitions: 10 each side

How Long to Hold: 2 seconds

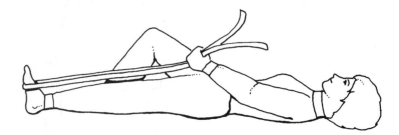

Lie on your back. Begin with your nonexercising knee bent and with that foot flat on the surface on which you are lying. Take your rope and hold the ends together so that it forms a loop. Place the foot of the leg you're exercising into the loop. Lock that knee so that your leg is extended straight out.

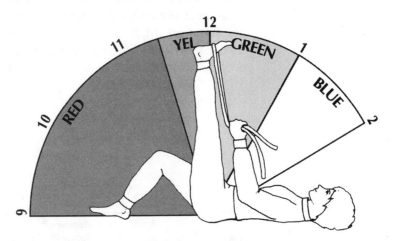

From your hip and using your quadriceps, lift your leg as far as you can. Aim your foot toward the ceiling. Grasp the ends of the rope (to maintain the loop) with both hands and "climb" up the rope, hand over hand, as your leg lifts. Keep slight tension on the rope. Use the rope for gentle assistance at the end of the stretch. Do not pull the leg into position or you will irritate the back of your knee.

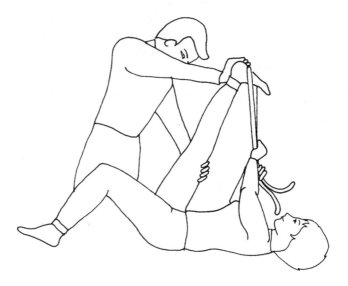

Assistant, help your athlete keep the knee locked. Let your athlete do all the work and use the rope, but provide gentle assistance at the end. Place one hand on the top of the thigh and one hand on the heel. Apply a little push for a 2-second hold. As the joint opens up, each successive stretch could be a little deeper, bringing the leg closer to the body.

Range	Position on Clock	Degree of Range of Motion
Red Range Too tight	9:00–11:30	0°–75°
Yellow Range Normal	11:30–12:00	75°–90°
Green Range Elite athlete	12:00–1:00	90°–120°
Blue Range Hypermobile	1:00–2:00	120°–150°

5 Hip Adductors

What You Stretch:	Muscles on the inside of the thigh (gracilis, adductor magnus, adductor longus and adductor brevis)
What You Contract:	Muscles on the outside of the thighs (abductors), muscles in the middle of your buttocks (gluteus medius), tensor fascia latae, and muscles that cross over the front thighs (sartorius)
How Many Repetitions:	10 each side
How Long to Hold:	2 seconds

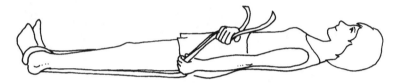

Lie on your back with both legs extended straight out. Take your rope and hold the ends together so that it forms a loop. Place the foot of the leg you're exercising into the loop and wrap the rope around the inside of the ankle so that the ends of the rope are on the outside. Lock that knee. Rotate your nonexercising leg inward slightly.

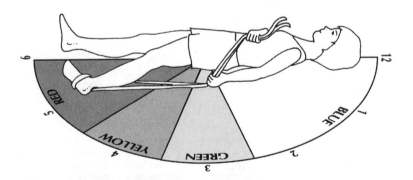

From your hip and using your abductors, extend your exercising leg out from the side of your body, leading with your heel. Keep slight tension on the rope. Use the rope for gentle assistance at the end of the stretch. Do not pull the leg into position and irritate your groin. Complete one set and then repeat, leading each stretch with the toe.

When Two Heads Are Better Than One . . .

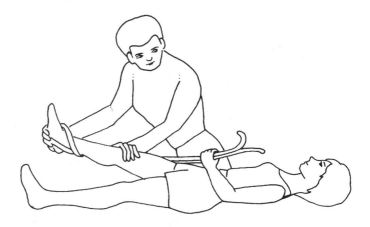

Assistant, help your athlete keep the knee locked. Let your athlete do all the work and use the rope, but provide gentle assistance at the end. Place one hand on the inside of the thigh and one hand on the heel. Apply a little pull for a 2-second hold. As the joint opens up, each successive stretch could be a little deeper.

Note: The starting position is with your feet at 6:00 on the clock face.

Left Side

Range	Position on Clock	Degree of Range of Motion
Red Range Too tight	6:00–4:30	0°–45°
Yellow Range Normal	4:30–3:30	45°–75°
Green Range Elite athlete	3:30–2:30	75°–105°
Blue Range Hypermobile	2:30–12:00	105°–180°

Right Side

Range	Position on Clock	Degree of Range of Motion
Red Range Too tight	6:00–7:30	0°–45°
Yellow Range Normal	7:30–8:30	45°–75°
Green Range Elite athlete	8:30–9:30	75°–105°
Blue Range Hypermobile	9:30–12:00	105°–180°

6   Hip Abductors

What You Stretch:	Muscles on the outside of the thighs/hips (gluteus medius, vastus lateralis, tensor fascia latae, and iliotibial band)
What You Contract:	Muscles on the inside of the thighs (gracilis, adductor magnus, adductor longus, and adductor brevis), pectinus, and quadriceps
How Many Repetitions:	10 each side
How Long to Hold:	2 seconds

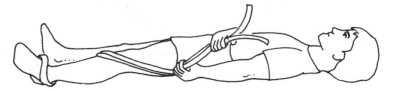

Lie on your back with both legs extended straight out. Take your rope and hold the ends together so that it forms a loop. Place the foot of the leg you're exercising into the loop and wrap the rope around the outside of the ankle so that the ends of the rope are on the inside. Lock that knee. Rotate your nonexercising leg inward slightly and rotate the exercising leg outward slightly. (They end up both pointing in the same direction.)

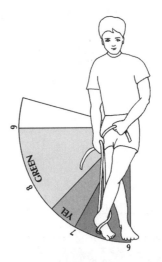

From your groin and using your adductors, extend your exercising leg across the midline of your body, leading with your heel just above the nonexercising leg. Keep slight tension on the rope. Use the rope for gentle assistance at the end of the stretch. Do not pull the leg into position or you will irritate your hip. Remember to keep your knee locked.

20

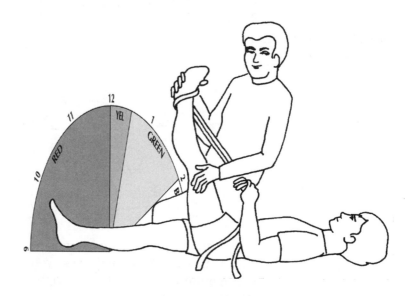

Assistant, help your athlete keep the knee locked and the exercising leg turned outward. Let your athlete do all the work and use the rope, but provide gentle assistance at the end. Place one hand on the outside of the thigh and one hand on the heel. Apply a little pull for a 2-second hold. As the joint opens up, each successive stretch could be a little deeper, bringing the leg farther across the body.

Note: The starting position is with your feet at 6:00 on the clock face.

Left Side

Range	Position on Clock	Degree of Range of Motion
Red Range Too tight	6:00–7:00	0°–30°
Yellow Range Normal	7:00–7:30	30°–45°
Green Range Elite athlete	7:30–9:00	45°–90°
Blue Range Hypermobile	9:00–9:15	90°–97.5°

Right Side

Range	Position on Clock	Degree of Range of Motion
Red Range Too tight	6:00–5:00	0°–30°
Yellow Range Normal	5:00–4:30	30°–45°
Green Range Elite athlete	4:30–3:00	45°–90°
Blue Range Hypermobile	3:00–2:45	90°–97.5°

21

7 Psoas

What You Stretch:	Muscles in the groin/front of upper thighs (the iliopsoas)
What You Contract:	Muscles in the buttocks (gluteus maximus) and back of thighs (hamstrings)
How Many Repetitions:	10 each side
How Long to Hold:	2 seconds

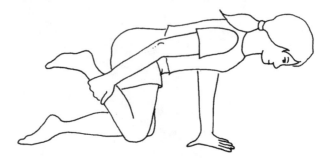

Position yourself on your hands and knees. Reach back with your right hand and grasp your right ankle. Reaching it will require that you lift your right foot to meet your hand. Hang on tightly.

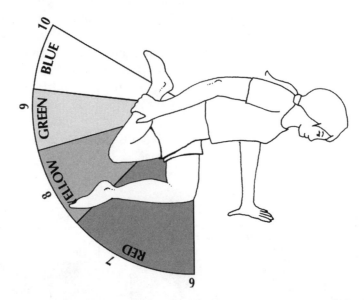

Using the hamstrings and the gluteus maximus, lift the exercising leg up until the thigh is parallel to the ground—or aligned horizontally with your body. Be careful not to arch your back (hyperextension). You may use your hand for gentle assistance at the end of the stretch.

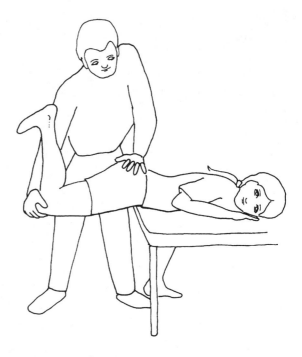

Assistant, stand behind your athlete. Cradle the exercising knee in your hand, bracing the shin against your forearm. Place your other hand on the buttock to keep the hips stable. Let your athlete do all the work, but provide gentle assistance at the end. Apply a little upward pull for a 2-second hold. As the joint opens up, each successive stretch could be a little deeper, bringing the leg higher.

Note: The starting position is with your knee at 6:00 on the clock face.

Range	Position on Clock	Degree of Range of Motion
Red Range Too tight	6:00–7:30	0°–45°
Yellow Range Normal	7:30–8:30	45°–75°
Green Range Elite athlete	8:30–9:15	75°–97.5°
Blue Range Hypermobile	9:15–10:00	97.5°–120°

8 Quadriceps

What You Stretch:	Muscles in the front of the thighs (rectus femoris)
What You Contract:	Muscles in the buttocks (gluteus maximus) and back of thighs (hamstrings)
How Many Repetitions:	10 each side
How Long to Hold:	2 seconds

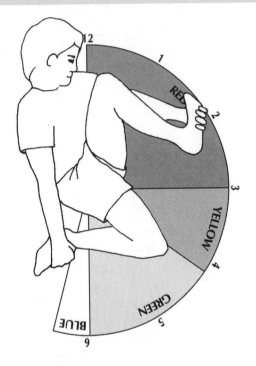

Lie on your side with your knees curled up against your chest (in a fetal position). Relax your neck, resting your head on the surface or on a pillow. Slide your bottom arm under the thigh of your bottom leg and place your hand around the outside of your foot. If you can't reach your foot, just stabilize your knee. Contract your abdominal muscles to keep from rolling. Reach down with your upper hand and grasp the shin (or ankle or forefoot) of your upper leg. If you are unable to bend your knee sufficiently for you to reach your foot with your hand, use your rope as an extender. Wrap it around your ankle and grasp the ends. Keep your knee bent and your leg parallel to the surface on which you are lying. Contract your hamstrings and gluteus maximus, and move that upper leg back as far as you can. You may use your hand to give a gentle assist at the end of the stretch.

When Two Heads Are Better Than One . . .

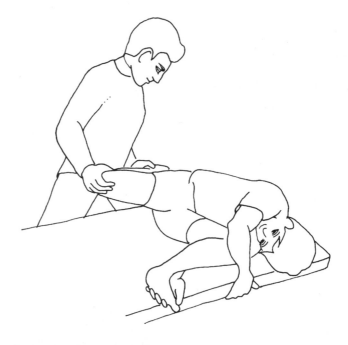

Assistant, let your athlete do all the work, but provide gentle assistance at the end. Apply a little pull for a 2-second hold. If your athlete is exceptionally tight, he or she can relax the knee and you can help bring the leg back and then bend the knee. Have the athlete contract the hamstrings to bring the heel to the buttocks. Assist with a gentle pull at the end, for a 2-second hold.

Note: View from above with head positioned at 12:00.

Left Side

Range	Position on Clock	Degree of Range of Motion
Red Range Too tight	12:00–9:00	0°–90°
Yellow Range Normal	9:00–7:45	90°–127.5°
Green Range Elite athlete	7:45–6:00	127.5°–180°
Blue Range Hypermobile	6:00–5:30	180°–195°

Right Side

Range	Position on Clock	Degree of Range of Motion
Red Range Too tight	12:00–3:00	0°–90°
Yellow Range Normal	3:00–4:15	90°–127.5°
Green Range Elite athlete	4:15–6:00	127.5°–180°
Blue Range Hypermobile	6:00–6:30	180°–195°

9 Gluteals

What You Stretch:	Lower back rotators, lateral hips, piriformis and buttocks (gluteus maximus)
What You Contract:	Abdominals, muscles from the front of the hips down the front of the thighs (hip flexors—including the quadriceps)
How Many Repetitions:	10 each side
How Long to Hold:	2 seconds

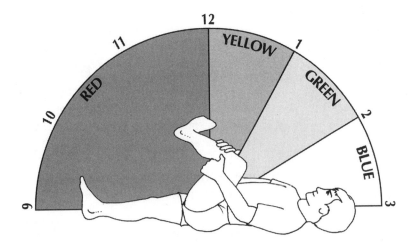

Lie flat on your back with both legs extended straight out. Rotate your nonexercising leg toward the midline of your body by pointing your toes inward. This stabilizes your hips. Using your abdominal muscles and hip flexors, lift your bent knee toward the opposite shoulder, keeping your pelvis flat on the surface. As your knee comes into range for easy reach, place your hand on the outside of your knee and gently guide the stretch. If you want a deeper stretch of the gluteus medius and piriformis, you can give your leg extra assistance by grasping the outside of your shin with the opposite hand and pressing your heel toward the floor as your knee nears your shoulder. Be careful that you do not irritate your knee.

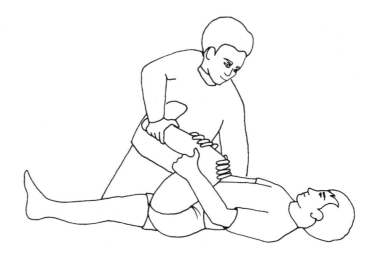

Assistant, let your athlete do all the work, but provide gentle assistance at the end. Place one hand on the top of the outside of the thigh and one hand on the ankle. Apply a little pull for a 2-second hold.

Note: View from above with head positioned at 3:00.

Range	Position on Clock	Degree of Range of Motion
Red Range Too tight	9:00–12:00	0°–90°
Yellow Range Normal	12:00–1:00	90°–120°
Green Range Elite athlete	1:00–2:00	120°–150°
Blue Range Hypermobile	2:00–3:00	150°–180°

10 Trunk Rotators

What You Stretch:	Lower back, midback muscles (erector spinae, deep posterior spinal group, and lumbar and thoracic spine rotators), and biceps femoris
What You Contract:	Muscles from the front of the hips down the front of the thighs (hip flexors—including the quadriceps), abdominals, and muscles on the inner thighs (adductors)
How Many Repetitions:	10 each side
How Long to Hold:	2 seconds

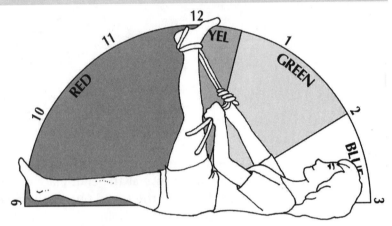

Note: It's important to maintain outward rotation of the exercising leg throughout the movement.

Lie on your back with both legs extended straight out. Take your rope and hold the ends together so that it forms a loop. Place the foot of the leg you're exercising into the loop and wrap the rope around the outside of the ankle. Draw the ends of the rope toward your inner thigh. Lock your knee. Rotate your nonexercising leg inward slightly and rotate the exercising leg outward slightly. (Your feet should be pointed in the same direction.) From your groin, and using your adductors, hip flexors, abdominals, and quadriceps, extend your exercising leg across the midline of your body. Aim your foot toward the opposite shoulder. Extend as far as you can go. Keep slight tension on the rope. Use the rope for gentle assistance at the end of the stretch. Do not pull the leg into position or you will irritate your hip. Remember to keep your knee locked.

Note: If muscles are exceptionally tight, start with non-exercising leg bent at a 90° angle with your foot on the surface.

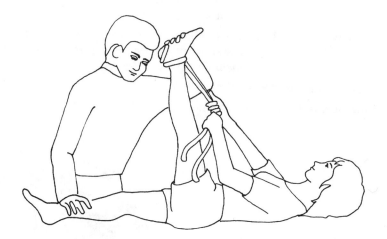

Assistant, help your athlete keep the knee locked. Let your athlete do all the work and use the rope, but provide gentle assistance at the end. Place one hand on the outer thigh above the knee and one hand on the heel. Apply a little pull for a 2-second hold. As the joint opens up, each successive stretch could be a little deeper, bringing the leg closer to the opposite shoulder.

Range	Position on Clock	Degree of Range of Motion
Red Range Too tight	9:00–12:00	0°–90°
Yellow Range Normal	12:00–12:30	90°–105°
Green Range Elite athlete	12:30–2:00	105°–150°
Blue Range Hypermobile	2:00–3:00	150°–180°

11   *Piriformis*

What You Stretch:	Muscles (piriformis) that lie underneath the big muscles (gluteus maximus) in the buttocks, low back rotators and external hip rotators
What You Contract:	Lower abdominals, hip rotators and adductors, and muscles from the front of the hips down the front of the thighs (hip flexors—including the quadriceps)
How Many Repetitions:	10 each side
How Long to Hold:	2 seconds

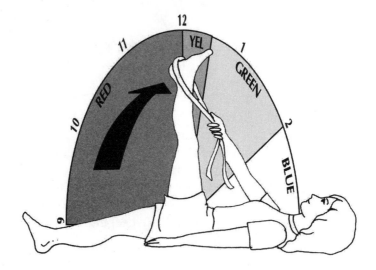

Lie on your back with both legs extended. Take your rope and hold the ends together so that it forms a loop. Place the foot of the leg you're exercising into the loop. Lock your knee so that your leg is straight. From your hip and using your quadriceps and hip flexors, lift your leg straight up until it is perpendicular to the surface (at a perfect 90° angle), "climbing" up the rope with both hands, hand over hand. Aim your foot toward the ceiling. When your leg is in position, grasp the ends of the rope (to maintain the loop) with the hand opposite the exercising leg. Extend your other hand (the one on the same side as the exercising leg) straight out to stabilize your body and keep you from rolling. Keep slight tension on the rope. Contract your adductors, internal hip rotators, and lower abdominals to bring your leg across your body and straight down to the surface until your hip begins to roll up. Use the rope for gentle assistance at the end of the stretch. Do not pull the leg into position or you will irritate your hip.

When Two Heads Are Better Than One . . .

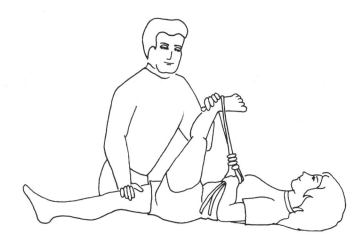

      Assistant, help your athlete keep the knee locked. Let your athlete do all the work and use the rope, but provide gentle assistance at the end. Place one hand on the heel of the exercising leg and one hand on the other thigh. Apply a little pull for a 2-second hold. As the joint opens up, each successive stretch could be a little deeper, bringing the foot of the exercising leg a little lower. It's important to keep your athlete from rolling, so maintain firm pressure on the thigh of the nonexercising leg.

Range	Position on Clock	Degree of Range of Motion
Red Range Too tight	9:00–10:00	0°–30°
Yellow Range Normal	10:00–10:30	30°–45°
Green Range Elite athlete	10:30–12:00	45°–90°
Blue Range Hypermobile	12:00–2:00	90°–120°

12 Hip External Rotators

What You Stretch:	The big muscles (gluteus maximus) in the buttocks and the deep external rotators (obturator externus, inferior and superior gemellus, obturator internus, and piriformis)
What You Contract:	The small muscles at the top of the buttocks toward the outside (gluteus minimus), the muscles that span from the hip sockets to the top of the pelvis (tensor fascia latae), and the muscles that attach from the bottom front of the pelvis to the inside of the thighs, halfway down the femurs (pectineus)
How Many Repetitions:	10 each side
How Long to Hold:	2 seconds

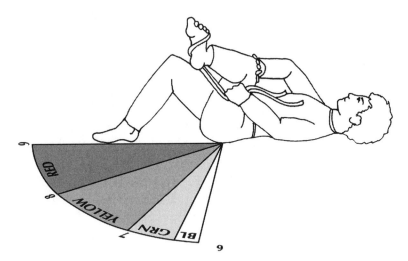

Lie on your back with your knees bent and your feet flat on the surface on which you are lying. Raise the foot of your exercising leg so that the thigh is at a 90° angle (your knee is at high noon) and the lower part of your leg is parallel to the surface. Take your rope and hold the ends together so that it forms a loop. Place the foot of the leg you're exercising into the loop. Wrap the ends of the rope around your ankle on the inside of the leg, and pull it under the bottom of your leg so that the hand on the same side as the exercising leg can grasp the ends of the rope. Place the other hand on the top of your thigh just at the knee, to stabilize and assist in rotation. Keeping the lower part of your leg parallel to the surface, rotate your thigh inward, pivoting your lower leg outward and leading with your heel. Your bracing hand and the rope may be used for a gentle assist at the end of the movement.

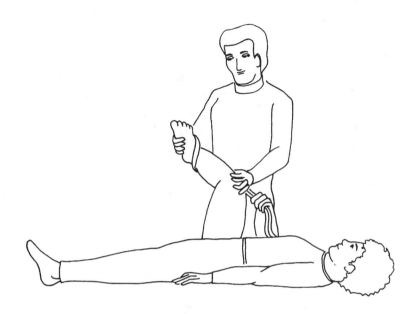

Assistant, let your athlete do all the work and use the rope, but provide gentle assistance at the end. Place one hand on the top of the thigh and one hand on the heel. Apply a little push for a 2-second hold. Use the hand on the thigh to assist in rotating the thigh so that the knee does not strain.

Left Side

Range	Position on Clock	Degree of Range of Motion
Red Range Too tight	12:00–11:00	0°–30°
Yellow Range Normal	11:00–10:00	30°–60°
Green Range Elite athlete	10:00–9:30	60°–75°
Blue Range Hypermobile	9:30–9:15	75°–82.5°

Right Side

Range	Position on Clock	Degree of Range of Motion
Red Range Too tight	12:00–1:00	0°–30°
Yellow Range Normal	1:00–2:00	30°–60°
Green Range Elite athlete	2:00–2:30	60°–75°
Blue Range Hypermobile	2:30–2:45	75°–82.5°

13 Hip Internal Rotators

What You Stretch:	The small muscles at the top of the buttocks toward the outside (gluteus minimus and medius), the muscles that span from the hip sockets to the top of the pelvis (tensor fascia latae), and the muscles that attach from the bottom front of the pelvis to the inside of the thighs, halfway down the femurs (pectineus)
What You Contract:	The big muscles (gluteus maximus) in the buttocks and the deep external rotators underneath (gemellus superior and inferior, obturator externus, quadratus femoris, and piriformis)
How Many Repetitions:	10 each side
How Long to Hold:	2 seconds

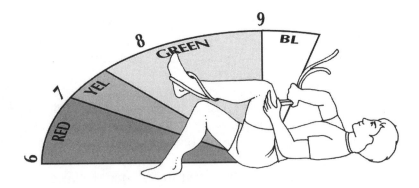

Lie on your back with your knees bent and your feet flat on the surface on which you are lying. Raise the foot of your exercising leg so the thigh is at a 90° angle (your knee is at high noon) and the lower part of your leg is parallel to the surface. Take your rope and hold the ends together so that it forms a loop. Place the foot of the leg you're exercising into the loop. Wrap the ends of the rope around your ankle on the outside of the leg, and pull it under the bottom of your leg so that the hand on the side opposite the exercising leg can grasp the ends of the rope. Place the other hand (on the same side as the exercising leg) on the top of your thigh just at the knee, to stabilize and assist in rotation. Keeping the lower part of your leg parallel to the surface, rotate your thigh outward, pivoting the lower part of your leg inward and leading with your heel. Your bracing hand and the rope may be used for a gentle assist at the end of the movement.

When Two Heads Are Better Than One . . .

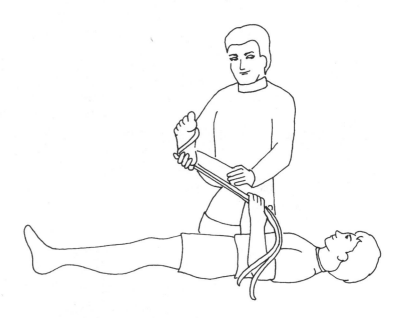

Assistant, let your athlete do all the work and use the rope, but provide gentle assistance at the end. Place one hand on the top of the thigh and one hand on the heel. Apply a little push for a 2-second hold. Use the hand on the thigh to assist in rotating the thigh so that the knee does not strain.

Left Side

Range	Position on Clock	Degree of Range of Motion
Red Range Too tight	6:00–7:00	0°–30°
Yellow Range Normal	7:00–7:30	30°–45°
Green Range Elite athlete	7:30–9:00	45°–90°
Blue Range Hypermobile	9:00–9:30	90°–105°

Right Side

Range	Position on Clock	Degree of Range of Motion
Red Range Too tight	6:00–5:00	0°–30°
Yellow Range Normal	5:00–4:30	30°–45°
Green Range Elite athlete	4:30–3:00	45°–90°
Blue Range Hypermobile	3:00–2:30	90°–105°

14 Medial Hip Rotators

What You Stretch:	The small muscles on the top of the buttocks toward the outside (gluteus minimus), the muscles that span from the hip sockets to the top of the pelvis (tensor fascia latae), the muscles that attach from the bottom front of the pelvis to the inside of the thighs, halfway down the femurs (pectineus), the muscles on the inside of the thighs (gracilis, adductor magnus, adductor longus, and adductor brevis), the muscles in the groin/front of the upper thighs (the iliopsoas), and the deep muscles on the inside of the pelvis that attach near the head of the femurs (iliacus)
What You Contract:	The big muscles (gluteus maximus) in the buttocks, the muscles in the middle of the buttocks (gluteus medius), and the deep external rotators underneath
How Many Repetitions:	10 each side
How Long to Hold:	2 seconds

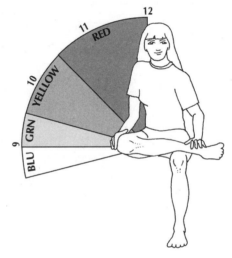

Note: You may want to use a folded towel on the top of your thigh, under the ankle of your exercising leg.

Sit in a chair with your back straight, or on a flat surface with your legs straight in front of you. The nonexercising leg is extended and locked at the knee. Take the foot of the leg to be exercised and place it on top of the thigh of the opposite leg, resting your ankle just over the knee. Contract the working muscles in your hip and outer thigh, and lower your knee as close to the surface as you can get. Using your nonexercising leg as a fulcrum, gently press your knee down with the hand on the same side, and stabilize and assist the stretch with your opposite hand by grasping your foot.

When Two Heads Are Better Than One . . .

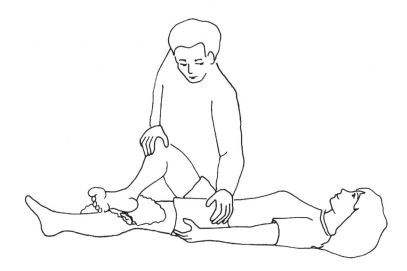

Assistant, when you assist, this exercise changes. The athlete is lying down on his or her back. Let your athlete do all the work, but provide gentle assistance at the end. Place one hand on the top of the pelvis at the hip bone and one hand on the inside of the knee of the exercising leg. Apply a little push for a 2-second hold. Use the hand on the pelvis to keep the athlete from raising the hip.

Left Side

Range	Position on Clock	Degree of Range of Motion
Red Range Too tight	12:00–1:30	0°–45°
Yellow Range Normal	1:30–2:30	45°–75°
Green Range Elite athlete	2:30–3:00	75°–90°
Blue Range Hypermobile	stopped by surface/floor	

Right Side

Range	Position on Clock	Degree of Range of Motion
Red Range Too tight	12:00–10:30	0°–45°
Yellow Range Normal	10:30–9:30	45°–75°
Green Range Elite athlete	9:30–9:00	75°–90°
Blue Range Hypermobile	stopped by surface/floor	

15 Trunk Extensors

What You Stretch:	The muscles that run from the pelvis to the base of the skull along the spine (erector spinae), and the back muscles below the belt line (sacrospinalis)
What You Contract:	Abdominals
How Many Repetitions:	10
How Long to Hold:	2 seconds

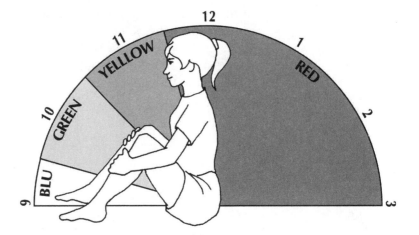

Sit with your back straight, your knees bent, your feet resting on your heels, and your toes pointed slightly up. Tuck your chin down, contract your abdominal muscles to pull your body forward. Grasp the sides of the lower legs with your hands to gently assist at the end of the stretch. To modify this exercise for a deeper lower-back stretch, bring your heels closer to your body and repeat the exercise.

When Two Heads Are Better Than One . . .

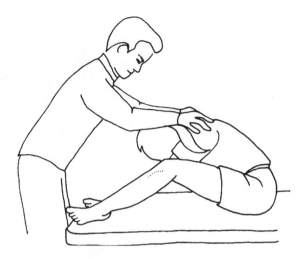

    Assistant, kneel in front of your athlete. Let your athlete do all the work, but provide gentle assistance at the end. Place your hands over his or her shoulder blades. Apply a little push for a 2-second hold.

Range	Position on Clock	Degree of Range of Motion
Red Range Too tight	3:00–11:30	0°–105°
Yellow Range Normal	11:30–10:30	105°–135°
Green Range Elite athlete	10:30–9:30	135°–165°
Blue Range Hypermobile	9:30–9:00	165°–180°

16 Thoracic-Lumbar Rotators

What You Stretch:	The muscles that run from the pelvis to the base of the skull along the spine (erector spinae), the muscles throughout your back and sides that stabilize your movement and help you to balance and change direction (thoracic-lumbar rotators), and the lower-back muscles below the belt line (sacrospinalis)
What You Contract:	Abdominals, the muscles on the sides of your chest (obliques), and the thoracic-lumbar rotators on the side opposite the exercising side
How Many Repetitions:	10 each side
How Long to Hold:	2 seconds

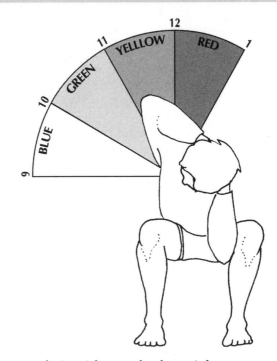

Sit in a chair with your back straight, or on a flat surface with your knees bent, your feet resting on your heels, and your toes pointed slightly up. Lock your hands behind your head, with your elbows out. Tuck your chin down. Contract your abdominal, oblique, and opposite thoracic-lumbar rotator muscles. Rotate your upper body in one direction until you have twisted as far as you can go. When you feel loosened up—after 4 or 5 repetitions in one direction—rotate, hold, and then flex your trunk forward, leading toward the ground with your elbow. Return to an upright position. Work one side at a time, completing all repetitions before beginning the opposite side.

When Two Heads Are Better Than One . . .

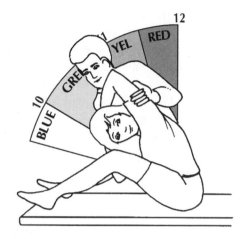

Assistant, let your athlete do all the work, but provide gentle assistance at the end. Place your hands on the side of the back just below the armpits. Apply a little twist for a 2-second hold. As the athlete lowers his or her upper body, you help maintain the rotation and assist in the downward move.

First Part: Rotation (Left Side)

Range	Position on Clock	Degree of Range of Motion
Red Range Too tight	3:00–2:00	0°–30°
Yellow Range Normal	2:00–1:00	30°–60°
Green Range Elite athlete	1:00–12:00	60°–90°
Blue Range Hypermobile	12:00–11:00	90°–120°

First Part: Rotation (Right Side)

Range	Position on Clock	Degree of Range of Motion
Red Range Too tight	9:00–10:00	0°–30°
Yellow Range Normal	10:00–11:00	30°–60°
Green Range Elite athlete	11:00–12:00	60°–90°
Blue Range Hypermobile	12:00–1:00	90°–120°

Second Part: Flexion While in Rotation

Range	Position on Clock	Degree of Range of Motion
Red Range Too tight	12:00–11:30	0°–15°
Yellow Range Normal	11:30–11:00	15°–30°
Green Range Elite athlete	11:00–10:00	30°–60°
Blue Range Hypermobile	10:00–9:30	60°–75°

17 Lateral Trunk Flexors

What You Stretch:	The muscles in your back along your spine, and the muscles in the sides of your trunk (lateral spine flexors, quadratus lumborum, obliques, and erector spinae)
What You Contract:	The muscles in your back along your spine, and the muscles in the sides of your trunk (lateral spine flexors, quadratus lumborum, obliques, and erector spinae) opposite the exercising side
How Many Repetitions:	10 each side
How Long to Hold:	2 seconds

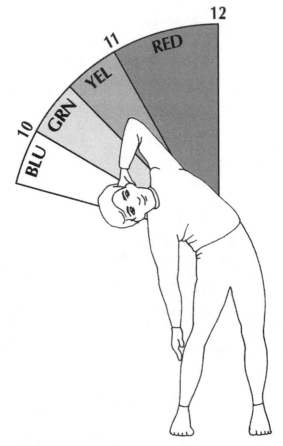

Stand with both arms at your sides. Raise one arm, placing that hand behind your head with the elbow pointed away from your body. Bend at the waist so that the arm that is straight is lowered down the side of the leg toward the knee and lower leg. This stretch can be modified by leaning slightly forward or backward before bending at the waist and lowering the arm down the side of the leg.

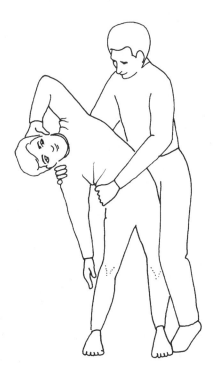

Assistant, stand behind your athlete. Let your athlete do all the work, but provide gentle assistance at the end. Place one hand on the shoulder and the other around the waist. Apply a little push at the shoulder for a 2-second hold.

Left Side

Range	Position on Clock	Degree of Range of Motion
Red Range Too tight	12:00–1:00	0°–30°
Yellow Range Normal	1:00–1:30	30°–45°
Green Range Elite athlete	1:30–2:00	45°–60°
Blue Range Hypermobile	2:00–2:30	60°–75°

Right Side

Range	Position on Clock	Degree of Range of Motion
Red Range Too tight	12:00–11:00	0°–30°
Yellow Range Normal	11:00–10:30	30°–45°
Green Range Elite athlete	10:30–10:00	45°–60°
Blue Range Hypermobile	10:00–9:30	60°–75°

Zone 2

Shoulders

18 *Shoulder Circumduction*

What You Stretch:	Nothing is specifically isolated. This is a gentle warm-up.
What You Contract:	Shoulders
How Many Repetitions:	10 each direction
How Long to Hold:	2 seconds

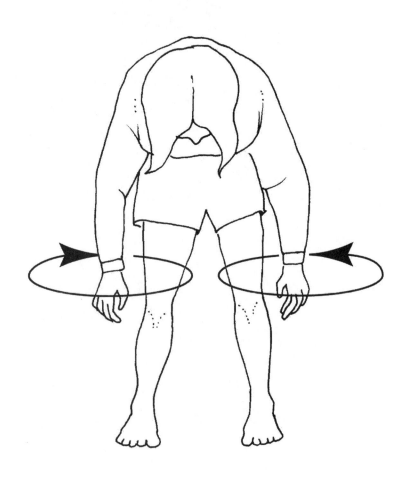

This stretch increases circulation in the shoulder joints (gleno-humeral joints). Stand, bending forward at the waist. Allow your arms to hang loosely. Bend your knees slightly to keep pressure off your back. Move your arms in small circles, allowing each arm to rotate from shoulder to hand. Move your arms clockwise and then counterclockwise. Start with small circles, then move to larger circles. Stay relaxed and keep your abdominal muscles tight.

Range	Position on Clock	Degree of Range of Motion
Red Range Too tight		
Yellow Range Normal		
Green Range Elite athlete		
Blue Range Hypermobile		

19 Pectoralis Major

What You Stretch:	Muscles in the chest and shoulders (pectoralis major, teres major, anterior deltoid)
What You Contract:	Backs of shoulders and area between the shoulder blades (trapezius, rhomboid major, and rhomboid minor)
How Many Repetitions:	10 each side
How Long to Hold:	2 seconds

This stretch is done in three progressive stages. The first reaching position has the arms below the belt. The second reaching position has the arms slightly level with the shoulders. And the last position has the arms above the shoulders.

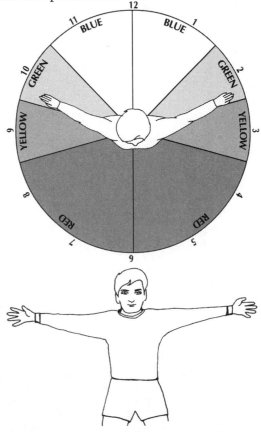

Stand with your feet slightly apart. Straighten your arms and lock your elbows. Face your palms forward so that your little finger is beside your thigh. Put your fingertips together in front of you and then swing both arms back (behind you), starting with the lowest position and progressing higher with each swing. Reach the highest level in ten repetitions.

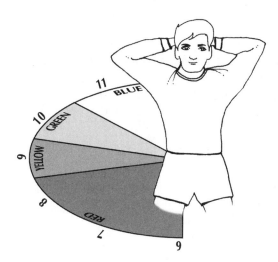

A modification of this stretch is to place your hands at the back of your head and touch your elbows in front of your face. Extend the elbows back as far as you can. Then return to the position where your elbows touch. This stretch isolates the outer attachment of the pectoralis major just under your collar bone.

When Two Heads Are Better Than One . . .

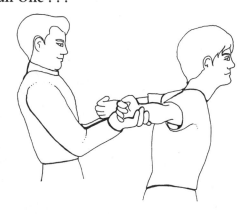

Assistant, stand behind your athlete. Let your athlete do all the work, but provide gentle assistance at the end. Grasp the wrists and apply a little pull for a 2-second hold.

Note: 0° = 6:00. Back of head is toward 12:00

Left Side

Range	Position on Clock	Degree of Range of Motion
Red Range Too tight	6:00–3:30	0°–75°
Yellow Range Normal	3:30–2:30	75°–105°
Green Range Elite athlete	2:30–1:30	105°–135°
Blue Range Hypermobile	1:30–12:00	135°–180°

Right Side

Range	Position on Clock	Degree of Range of Motion
Red Range Too tight	6:00–8:30	0°–75°
Yellow Range Normal	8:30–9:30	75°–105°
Green Range Elite athlete	9:30–10:30	105°–135°
Blue Range Hypermobile	10:30–12:00	135°–180°

20 *Anterior Deltoid*

What You Stretch:	Upper arms and shoulders (biceps brachii and anterior deltoid), pectoralis major and minor
What You Contract:	Back of shoulders, triceps, and posterior deltoids
How Many Repetitions:	10
How Long to Hold:	2 seconds

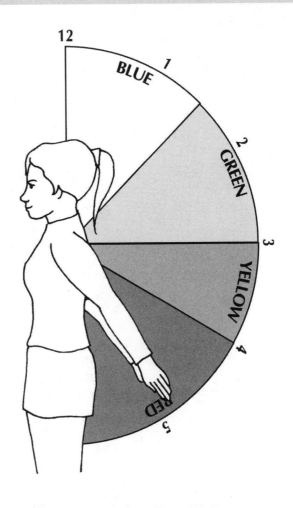

Stand with your feet slightly apart and your arms loosely by your sides. Begin to reach backward with your arms, keeping your elbows locked and your palms facing backward. Loosen up with about ten repetitions. To modify this exercise for a deeper stretch, touch your fingers together. Continue reaching backward, keeping your elbows locked and raising your arms slightly to achieve the stretch.

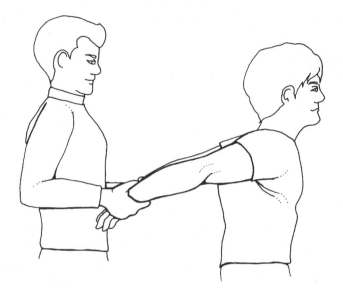

Zone 2

Assistant, stand behind your athlete. Let your athlete do all the work, but provide gentle assistance at the end. Grasp the wrists and apply a little pull for a 2-second hold.

Range	Position on Clock	Degree of Range of Motion
Red Range Too tight	6:00–4:00	0°–60°
Yellow Range Normal	4:00–3:00	60°–90°
Green Range Elite athlete	3:00–1:30	90°–135°
Blue Range Hypermobile	1:30–12:00	135°–180°

21 *Shoulder Internal Rotators*

What You Stretch:	Internal rotator muscles in the shoulder (teres major, subscapularis, and pectoralis major)
What You Contract:	External rotator muscles in the back of your shoulders (supraspinatus, infraspinatus, teres minor)
How Many Repetitions:	10 each side
How Long to Hold:	2 seconds

Stand with your feet slightly apart. Raise your arms to shoulder level, with the upper part of your arms horizontal to your shoulders. Bend your elbows so that your forearms and hands are in front of your body. Your palms should be facing down. Rotate your forearms and hands up and back, extending as far as you can beyond the midline of your body.

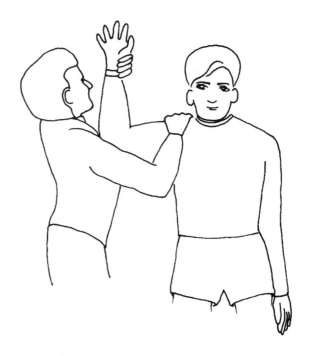

Zone 2

Assistant, let your athlete do all the work, but provide gentle assistance at the end. Place one hand over the athlete's shoulder from the front. Grasp the exercising forearm at the wrist with your other hand. Stabilize the elbow on your chest. Apply a little push for a 2-second hold.

Note: Athlete faces 3:00 or 0°.

Range	Position on Clock	Degree of Range of Motion
Red Range Too tight	3:00–12:00	0°–90°
Yellow Range Normal	12:00–11:30	90°–105°
Green Range Elite athlete	11:30–10:30	105°–135°
Blue Range Hypermobile	10:30–9:30	135°–165°

22 *Shoulder External Rotators*

What You Stretch:	External rotator muscles in the back of your shoulders (supraspinatus, infraspinatus, teres minor)
What You Contract:	Internal rotator muscles in the shoulders (teres major, subscapularis, and pectoralis major)
How Many Repetitions:	10 each side
How Long to Hold:	2 seconds

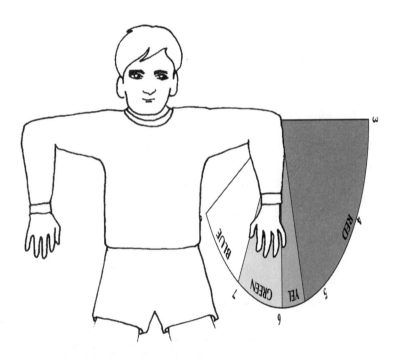

Stand with your feet slightly apart. Raise your arms to shoulder level, with the upper part of your arm horizontal to your shoulders. Bend your elbows so that your forearms and hands are in front of your body. Your palms should be facing down. Rotate your forearms and hands down and back, extending as far as you can beyond the midline of your body. Keep your elbow at shoulder height and keep your shoulders level.

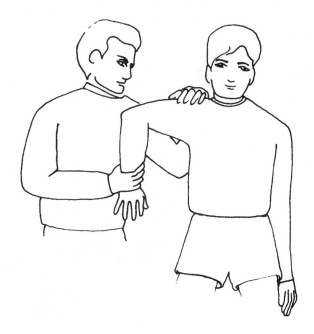

Assistant, let your athlete do all the work, but provide gentle assistance at the end. Place one hand over the athlete's shoulder from the back. Clamp down and pull back. Grasp the wrist of the exercising forearm in the other hand. Stabilize the elbow on your shoulder. Apply a little pull for a 2-second hold.

Note: Athlete faces 9:00 or 0°.

Range	Position on Clock	Degree of Range of Motion
Red Range Too tight	3:00–5:30	0°–75°
Yellow Range Normal	5:30–6:00	75°–90°
Green Range Elite athlete	6:00–7:00	90°–120°
Blue Range Hypermobile	7:00–8:00	120°–150°

23 Rhomboid/Rotator Cuff

What You Stretch:	External shoulder rotators—commonly called the rotator cuff (supraspinatus, infraspinatus and teres minor), and rhomboid major and minor
What You Contract:	Muscles in the shoulder (pectoralis major, anterior deltoid, and coracobrachialis)
How Many Repetitions:	10 each side
How Long to Hold:	2 seconds

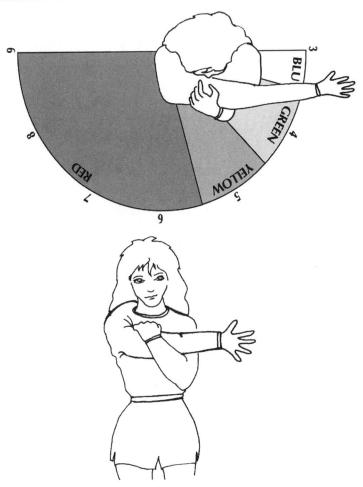

Stand with your feet slightly apart and your arms at your sides. Lift one arm, with the elbow locked, and raise it across your chest toward the opposite shoulder. Use the other hand to give a gentle assist at the elbow, at the end of the movement. Keep your torso still, and resist the temptation to "hike" up your shoulder.

When Two Heads Are Better Than One . . .

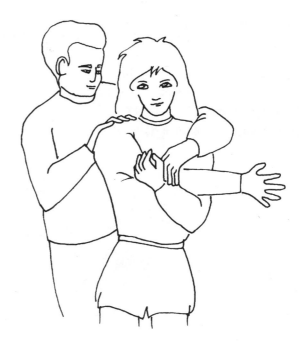

Assistant, let your athlete do all the work, but provide gentle assistance at the end. Place one hand over the athlete's shoulder from the back. Press down. Grasp the exercising elbow in the other hand. Apply a little pull for a 2-second hold.

Note: Athlete faces 6:00. 0° = 9:00.

Left Side

Range	Position on Clock	Degree of Range of Motion
Red Range Too tight	3:00–6:30	0°–105°
Yellow Range Normal	6:30–7:30	105°–135°
Green Range Elite athlete	7:30–8:30	135°–165°
Blue Range Hypermobile	8:30–9:00	165°–180°

Right Side

Range	Position on Clock	Degree of Range of Motion
Red Range Too tight	9:00–5:30	0°–105°
Yellow Range Normal	5:30–4:30	105°–135°
Green Range Elite athlete	4:30–3:30	135°–165°
Blue Range Hypermobile	3:30–3:00	165°–180°

24 *Trapezius/Rotator Cuff*

What You Stretch:	External shoulder rotators—commonly called the rotator cuffs (teres minor, infraspinatus), muscles below the shoulder blades (latissimus dorsi), and trapezius
What You Contract:	Muscles in the shoulders (pectoralis major, anterior deltoid, and coracobrachialis)
How Many Repetitions:	10 each side
How Long to Hold:	2 seconds

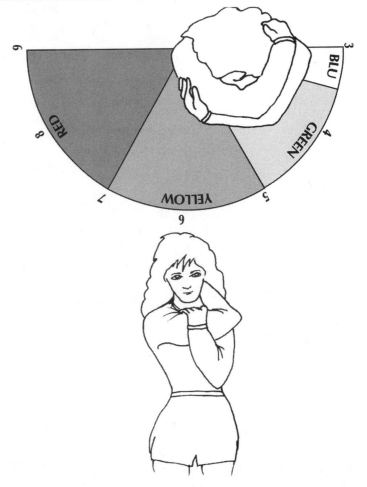

Stand with your feet slightly apart and your arms at your sides. Lift one arm, with the elbow bent, and raise it across your chest over the opposite shoulder until your hand reaches down your back. Use the other hand to give a gentle assist at the elbow, at the end of the movement. Keep your torso still, and resist the temptation to "hike" up your shoulder.

When Two Heads Are Better Than One . . .

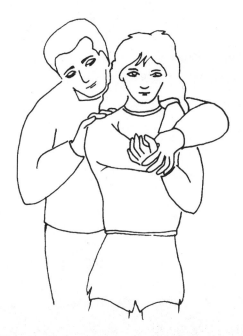

Assistant, let your athlete do all the work, but provide gentle assistance at the end. Place one hand over the athlete's shoulder from the back. Grasp the exercising elbow in the other hand. Apply a little pull for a 2-second hold.

Note: 0° = 9:00.

Left Side

Range	Position on Clock	Degree of Range of Motion
Red Range Too tight	3:00–5:00	0°–60°
Yellow Range Normal	5:00–7:00	60°–120°
Green Range Elite athlete	7:00–8:30	120°–165°
Blue Range Hypermobile	8:30–9:00	165°–180°

Right Side

Range	Position on Clock	Degree of Range of Motion
Red Range Too tight	9:00–7:00	0°–60°
Yellow Range Normal	7:00–5:00	60°–120°
Green Range Elite athlete	5:00–3:30	120°–165°
Blue Range Hypermobile	3:30–3:00	165°–180°

25 Forward Elevation of the Shoulder

What You Stretch:	Muscles in the shoulders (supraspinatus, infraspinatus, teres minor, teres major, subscapularis, and pectoralis major), upper triceps, serratus anterior, and posterior deltoid
What You Contract:	Muscles in the shoulders (upper biceps brachii and anterior deltoid)
How Many Repetitions:	10 each side
How Long to Hold:	2 seconds

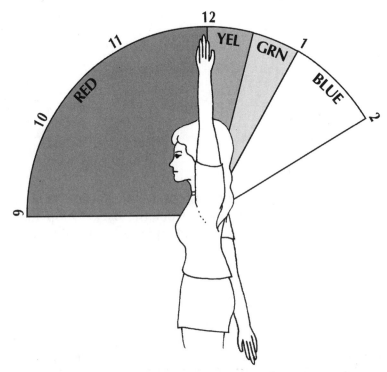

Stand with your feet slightly apart and your arms by your sides. Raise one arm, with the elbow locked, above your head. Working in opposition, with equal resistance, extend your nonexercising arm behind you. Your palms should face in toward the center line of your body. The movement looks like the arm action of a marching tin soldier. After several repetitions, face your palms forward. After several more repetitions, face your palms outward.

When Two Heads Are Better Than One . . .

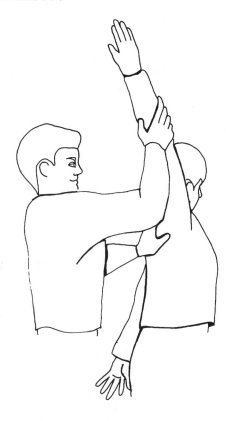

Assistant, stand behind your athlete. Let your athlete do all the work, but provide gentle assistance at the end. Grasp the upraised arm just above the elbow. Brace with the other hand on the shoulder blade. Apply a little pull for a 2-second hold.

Note: 0° = 9:00.

Range	Position on Clock	Degree of Range of Motion
Red Range Too tight	9:00–12:00	0°–90°
Yellow Range Normal	12:00–12:30	90°–105°
Green Range Elite athlete	12:30–1:00	105°–120°
Blue Range Hypermobile	1:00–2:00	120°–150°

26 Sideways Elevation of the Shoulder

Zone 2

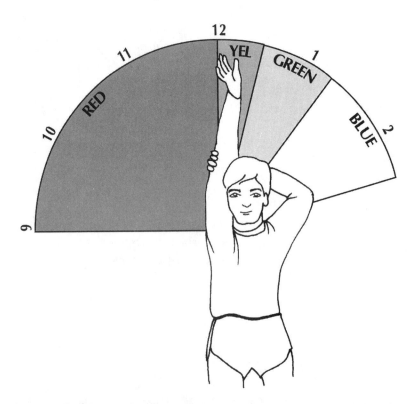

Stand with your feet slightly apart and your arms by your sides. Bend your knees and tighten your abdominals. With your elbow locked and the palm facing forward, raise one arm above and behind your head. Using the nonexercising hand, reach over and grasp the exercising arm between the elbow and shoulder. Gently assist the stretch until you feel a pull at the base of your shoulder blade.

When Two Heads Are Better Than One . . .

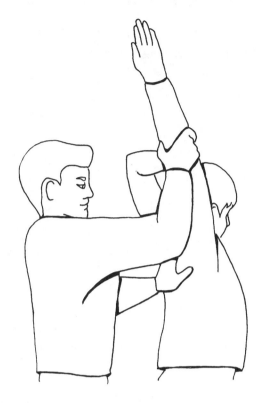

Assistant, stand behind your athlete. Let your athlete do all the work, but provide gentle assistance at the end. Grasp the arm just above the elbow. Brace with the other hand on the shoulder blade. Apply a little push for a 2-second hold.

Note: Right side: 0° = 9:00. Left side: 0° = 3:00.

Left Side

Range	Position on Clock	Degree of Range of Motion
Red Range Too tight	3:00–12:00	0°–90°
Yellow Range Normal	12:00–11:30	90°–105°
Green Range Elite athlete	11:30–10:30	105°–135°
Blue Range Hypermobile	10:30–9:30	135°–165°

Right Side

Range	Position on Clock	Degree of Range of Motion
Red Range Too tight	9:00–12:00	0°–90°
Yellow Range Normal	12:00–12:30	90°–105°
Green Range Elite athlete	12:30–1:30	105°–135°
Blue Range Hypermobile	1:30–2:30	135°–165°

27 Posterior Hand Clasp

What You Stretch:	Muscles in the shoulders (all)
What You Contract:	Muscles in the shoulders (all)
How Many Repetitions:	10 each side
How Long to Hold:	2 seconds

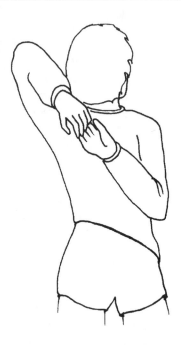

This is not so much an Active-Isolated Stretch as it is a "test" that allows you to determine your success in opening up your shoulder. Stand with your feet slightly apart and your arms at your sides. Bend your knees slightly. Raise one arm, bend it at the elbow, and reach down until your hand is between the shoulder blades of the upper back. With the other arm bent at the elbow, reach behind the back until your fingertips touch the hand that is down between the shoulder blades. If possible, clasp your fingers and gently stretch. You can use a stretch rope to connect your hands behind your back. "Climb" up or down the rope to assist the stretch and gain a little range of motion. Interestingly, most people are more flexible on one side than the other. How do you know that you have done well? If you cannot touch, then you have work to do. If you can just touch fingertips, you're making progress, but you are not yet in full range of motion. If you can clasp hands, shake your own hand. You've done well.

When Two Heads Are Better Than One . . .

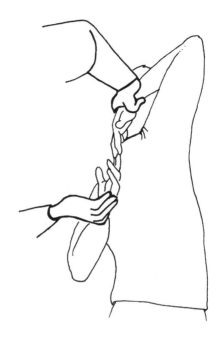

Zone 2

Assistant, stand behind your athlete. Let your athlete do all the work, but provide gentle assistance at the end. Grasp the wrists. Apply a little pull for a 2-second hold.

Range	Position on Clock	Degree of Range of Motion
Red Range Too tight		
Yellow Range Normal		
Green Range Elite athlete		
Blue Range Hypermobile		

Zone 3

Neck

28 Neck Semi-Circumduction

What You Stretch:	Nothing specifically isolated. This is a gentle warm-up
What You Contract:	Neck
How Many Repetitions:	10 in each direction
How Long to Hold:	2 seconds

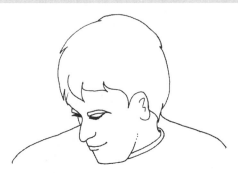

This two-part exercise increases circulation in the neck. Sit with your hands on your knees. The first part of this exercise is to face forward and then turn your head to the side, looking over one shoulder. Relax your neck, allowing your head to roll gently toward the midline of your body until your chin is against your chest. Continue the gentle roll until your head is back up over the opposite shoulder and you are looking over that shoulder. Allow your head to fall forward again and roll back the other way. The second part of this exercise is to face forward and then turn your head to the side, looking over one shoulder. Relax your neck, allowing your head to roll gently backward. Continue to roll your head toward the opposite shoulder, hyperextending your neck as much as you comfortably can. When you reach the opposite shoulder, roll your head back the other way.

Range	Position on Clock	Degree of Range of Motion
Red Range Too tight		
Yellow Range Normal		
Green Range Elite athlete		
Blue Range Hypermobile		

29 Neck Extensors

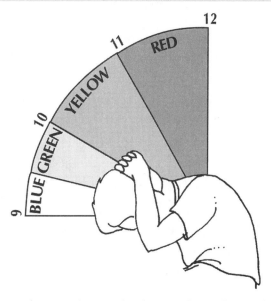

Sit in a chair with your back straight and your feet flat on the floor. With your hands placed on the back of your head, tuck your chin and roll your head forward until your chin meets your chest. You can gently assist the end of the movement with your hands at the back of your head. Be certain to keep your shoulders down.

Note: 0° = 12:00.

Range	Position on Clock	Degree of Range of Motion
Red Range Too tight	12:00–11:00	0°–30°
Yellow Range Normal	11:00–10:00	30°–60°
Green Range Elite athlete	10:00–9:30	60°–75°
Blue Range Hypermobile	9:30–9:00	75°–90°

Zone 3

30 Neck Flexors

What You Stretch:	Muscles in the front of the neck (anterior cervical flexor muscles)
What You Contract:	Muscles in the back of the neck (cervical extensors) and the top of the back (erector spinae)
How Many Repetitions:	10
How Long to Hold:	2 seconds

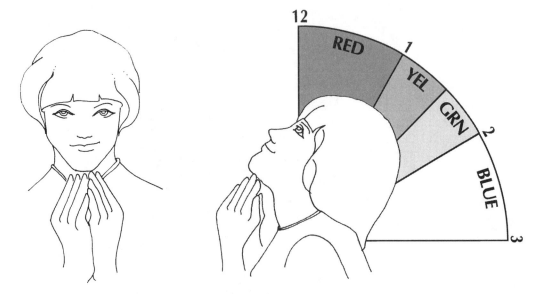

Sit in a chair with your back straight and your feet flat on the floor. Place your fingertips along your jaw line just under your chin and roll your head backward very gently. You can gently assist the end of the movement with your fingertips. Be certain to keep your shoulders down.

Note: 0° = 12:00.

Range	Position on Clock	Degree of Range of Motion
Red Range Too tight	12:00–1:00	0°–30°
Yellow Range Normal	1:00–1:30	30°–45°
Green Range Elite athlete	1:30–2:00	45°–60°
Blue Range Hypermobile	2:00–3:00	60°–90°

31 Neck Lateral Flexors

What You Stretch:	Muscles in the side of the neck (cervical lateral flexors)
What You Contract:	Muscles in the opposite side of the neck (cervical lateral flexors)
How Many Repetitions:	10 each side
How Long to Hold:	2 seconds

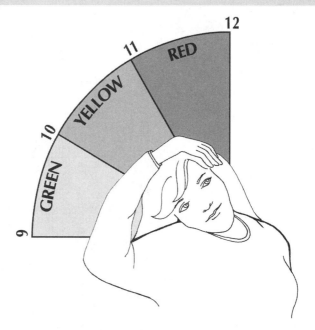

Sit in a chair with your back straight and your feet flat on the floor. Look straight ahead. "Cock" your head to one side, lowering your ear straight down toward your shoulder. Reach up over the top of your head with the hand that is on the same side as the shoulder, gently place your fingertips on your temple, and press very gently down, to assist the end of the movement. Be certain to keep your shoulders down and your body still.

Left Side

Range	Position on Clock	Degree of Range of Motion
Red Range Too tight	12:00–1:00	0°–30°
Yellow Range Normal	1:00–2:00	30°–60°
Green Range Elite athlete	2:00–3:00	60°–90°
Blue Range Hypermobile	(Head stops at shoulder)	

Right Side

Range	Position on Clock	Degree of Range of Motion
Red Range Too tight	12:00–11:00	0°–30°
Yellow Range Normal	11:00–10:00	30°–60°
Green Range Elite athlete	10:00–9:00	60°–90°
Blue Range Hypermobile	(Head stops at shoulder)	

Zone 3

71

32 Neck Rotators

What You Stretch:	Muscles in the side of the neck (cervical rotators)
What You Contract:	Muscles in the opposite side of the neck (cervical rotators)
How Many Repetitions:	10 each side
How Long to Hold:	2 seconds

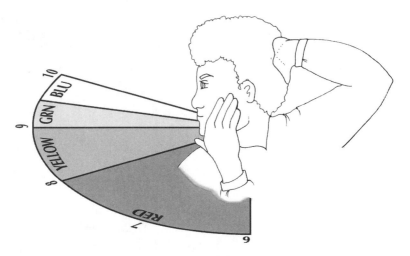

Sit on a chair with your back straight and your feet flat on the floor. Look straight ahead. Turn your head to one side until your chin is over your shoulder. If you're turning to the right, reach up with your left hand and place it behind your head at the base of the skull. Apply gentle pressure to assist the end of the movement. Take your right hand and place the fingertips along your left jawline. Press very gently to guide the end of the stretch. Be certain to keep your shoulders down and your body still. Turn your head to the other side and repeat the stretch.

Note: 0° = 6:00.

Left Side

Range	Position on Clock	Degree of Range of Motion
Red Range Too tight	6:00–4:00	0°–60°
Yellow Range Normal	4:00–3:00	60°–90°
Green Range Elite athlete	3:00–2:30	90°–105°
Blue Range Hypermobile	2:30–2:00	105°–120°

Right Side

Range	Position on Clock	Degree of Range of Motion
Red Range Too tight	6:00–8:00	0°–60°
Yellow Range Normal	8:00–9:00	60°–90°
Green Range Elite athlete	9:00–9:30	90°–105°
Blue Range Hypermobile	9:30–10:00	105°–120°

33 Neck Oblique Extensors

What You Stretch:	Muscles in the upper shoulders at the base of the neck (including the trapezius)
What You Contract:	Muscles in the front of the neck (cervical flexors)
How Many Repetitions:	10 each side
How Long to Hold:	2 seconds

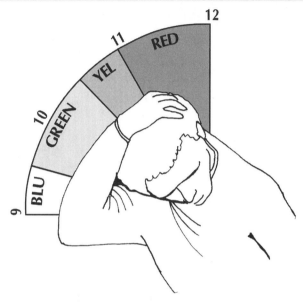

Sit in a chair with your back straight and your feet flat on the floor. Turn your head right to a 45° angle. Then, drop your head forward, bringing your right ear toward your chest. Place your left hand on top of your head and gently press down to assist the end of the movement. Be certain to keep your shoulders down and your body still.

Note: 0° = 12:00.

Left Side

Range	Position on Clock	Degree of Range of Motion
Red Range Too tight	12:00–1:00	0°–30°
Yellow Range Normal	1:00–1:30	30°–45°
Green Range Elite athlete	1:30–2:30	45°–75°
Blue Range Hypermobile	2:30–3:00	75°–90°

Right Side

Range	Position on Clock	Degree of Range of Motion
Red Range Too tight	12:00–11:00	0°–30°
Yellow Range Normal	11:00–10:30	30°–45°
Green Range Elite athlete	10:30–9:30	45°–75°
Blue Range Hypermobile	9:30–9:00	75°–90°

34 *Neck Oblique Flexors*

What You Stretch:	Muscles in the neck (cervical flexors, especially the three scalenus muscles)
What You Contract:	Muscles in the base of the neck (cervical extensors)
How Many Repetitions:	10 each side
How Long to Hold:	2 seconds

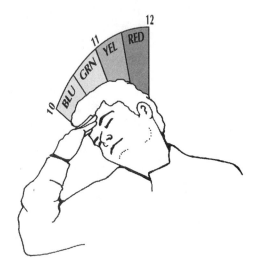

Sit in a chair with your back straight and your feet flat on the floor. Turn your head right to a 45° angle. Then, drop your head backward, bringing your ear toward your shoulder. Place your right hand on your forehead and gently press back to assist the end of the movement. Be certain to keep your shoulders down and keep your body still.

Note: 0° = 12:00.

Left Side

Range	Position on Clock	Degree of Range of Motion
Red Range Too tight	12:00–12:30	0°–15°
Yellow Range Normal	12:30–1:00	15°–30°
Green Range Elite athlete	1:00–1:30	30°–45°
Blue Range Hypermobile	1:30–2:00	45°–60°

Right Side

Range	Position on Clock	Degree of Range of Motion
Red Range Too tight	12:00–11:30	0°–15°
Yellow Range Normal	11:30–11:00	15°–30°
Green Range Elite athlete	11:00–10:30	30°–45°
Blue Range Hypermobile	10:30–10:00	45°–60°

Zone 4

Arms, Elbows, Wrists, and Hands

35 Elbow Flexors

What You Stretch:	Muscles in the front of the upper arms (biceps brachii, brachialis, brachioradialis)
What You Contract:	Muscles in the back of the upper arms (triceps brachii), and muscles on the inside of the forearm (posterior radio-ulnar extensors)
How Many Repetitions:	10 each side
How Long to Hold:	2 seconds

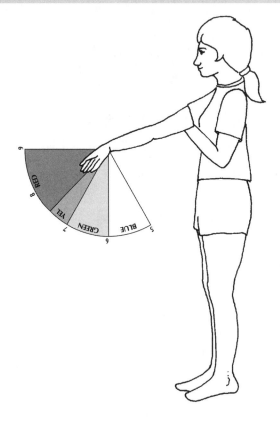

Zone 4

Note: This exercise also can be done while sitting in a chair.

Stand with your feet a few inches apart and slightly bend your knees. Drop your exercising arm straight by your side and then flex your elbow until your forearm is parallel with the floor and your palm is facing your body (inward) with your thumb up. Reach across your body with your nonexercising arm, and rest the elbow of your exercising arm in the palm of your hand. Holding your upper arm still, extend the exercising arm from the elbow down toward the floor until it's as straight as possible. Lock your fingers straight with your palm still turned inward. At the end of the movement, continue flexing your wrist by following your little finger straight back. You'll feel the stretch in the top of your lower arm from your thumb to your elbow.

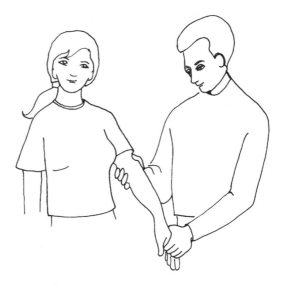

Assistant, stand beside your athlete. Support the elbow. Grasp your athlete's hand as if you were "shaking hands." Let your athlete do all the work, but apply a gentle downward press for a 2-second hold.

Note: 0° = 9:00.

Zone 4

Range	Position on Clock	Degree of Range of Motion
Red Range Too tight	9:00–7:30	0°–45°
Yellow Range Normal	7:30–7:00	45°–60°
Green Range Elite athlete	7:00–6:00	60°–90°
Blue Range Hypermobile	6:00–5:30	90°–105°

36 Biceps

What You Stretch:	Muscles in the front of the upper arms (biceps brachii, brachialis, brachio-radialis)
What You Contract:	Muscles in the back of the upper arms (triceps brachii, posterior deltoids, and the posterior radio-ulnar extensors)
How Many Repetitions:	10
How Long to Hold:	2 seconds

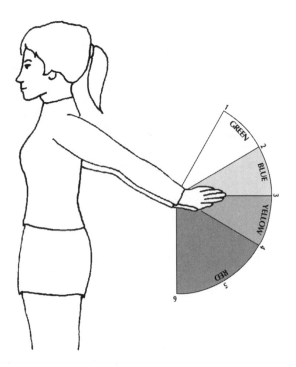

Note: This exercise can be done while sitting on a chair.

Stand with your feet a few inches apart, and slightly bend your knees. Put your arms at your sides, with the elbow of your exercising arm locked. Leading with your little finger, swing the exercising arm straight back behind you. Keep your palm facing in, and flex the wrist at the end of the motion, to point your hand upward.

Zone 4

78

When Two Heads Are Better Than One . . .

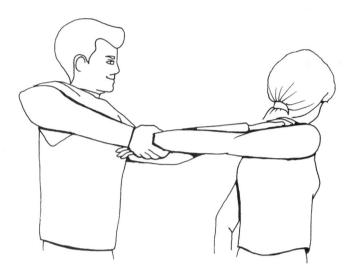

    Assistant, stand behind your athlete. Let your athlete do all the work, but provide gentle assistance at the end. Grasp the wrist of the exercising arm. Brace with the other hand on the shoulder blade. Apply a little lift for a 2-second hold.

Note: 0° = 6:00.

Range	Position on Clock	Degree of Range of Motion
Red Range Too tight	6:00–4:00	0°–60°
Yellow Range Normal	4:00–3:00	60°–90°
Green Range Elite athlete	3:00–2:00	90°–120°
Blue Range Hypermobile	2:00–1:00	120°–150°

37 Triceps

What You Stretch:	Muscles in the back of your upper arms (triceps brachii)
What You Contract:	Muscles in the front of your upper arms (biceps brachii and anterior deltoids)
How Many Repetitions:	10 each side
How Long to Hold:	2 seconds

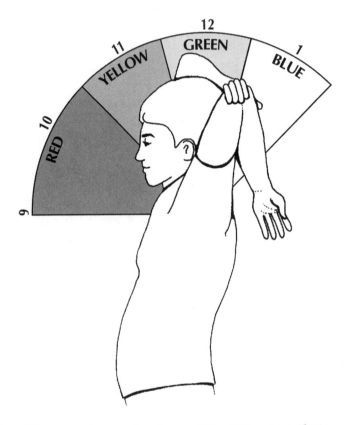

Note: This exercise can be done while sitting in a chair.

Stand with your feet a few inches apart and slightly bend your knees. Lift the exercising arm, with elbow bent, and raise it until your hand reaches over your shoulder and down your back. Use the other hand to give a gentle assist at the elbow, at the end of the movement. Keep your torso still and your back straight, and resist the temptation to "hike" up your shoulder.

Zone 4

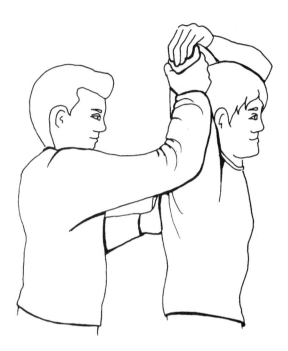

Assistant, stand behind your athlete. Let your athlete do all the work, but provide gentle assistance at the end. Grasp the elbow of the exercising arm. Brace with the other hand on the shoulder blade. Apply a little lift and backward push for a 2-second hold.

Note: 0° = 9:00.

Zone 4

Range	Position on Clock	Degree of Range of Motion
Red Range Too tight	9:00–10:30	0°–45°
Yellow Range Normal	10:30–11:30	45°–75°
Green Range Elite athlete	11:30–12:30	75°–105°
Blue Range Hypermobile	12:30–1:30	105°–135°

38 Radio-Ulnar Supinators

What You Stretch:	Muscles in the upper arms (supinator brevis and the lower attachment of the biceps brachii)
What You Contract:	Muscles in the lower arms (pronator quadratus and the pronator teres)
How Many Repetitions:	10 each side
How Long to Hold:	2 seconds

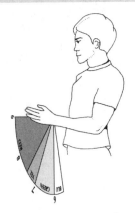 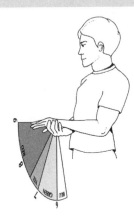

Note: This exercise also can be done while sitting in a chair.

Stand with your feet a few inches apart and slightly bend your knees. Drop your nonexercising arm by your side and bend the exercising arm at the elbow until your forearm is extending straight out from your body. Keep the bent elbow close to your side with your palm facing downward. Reach across with the nonexercising hand and place its palm over the back of the hand on the exercising arm. Wrap the fingers of the non-exercising hand around the back of the exercising hand between the base of the little finger and the wrist. Grasp gently. Without assisting, twist your exercising wrist so that the palm faces outward and your thumb leads to the floor. You'll feel the stretch in your forearm. You may assist the end of the movement with your nonexercising hand.

Note: Right hand: 0° = 3:00. Left hand: 0° = 9:00.

Left Side

Range	Position on Clock	Degree of Range of Motion
Red Range Too tight	9:00–7:30	0°–45°
Yellow Range Normal	7:30–7:00	45°–60°
Green Range Elite athlete	7:00–6:00	60°–90°
Blue Range Hypermobile	6:00–5:30	90°–105°

Right Side

Range	Position on Clock	Degree of Range of Motion
Red Range Too tight	3:00–4:30	0°–45°
Yellow Range Normal	4:30–5:00	45°–60°
Green Range Elite athlete	5:00–6:00	60°–90°
Blue Range Hypermobile	6:00–6:30	90°–105°

Zone 4

39 Radio-Ulnar Pronators

What You Stretch:	Muscles in the lower arms (pronator quadratus and the pronator teres)
What You Contract:	Muscles in the upper arms (supinator brevis and the lower attachment of the biceps brachii)
How Many Repetitions:	10 each side
How Long to Hold:	2 seconds

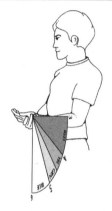 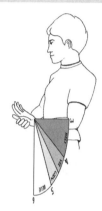

Note: This exercise also can be done while sitting on a chair.

Stand with your feet a few inches apart and slightly bend your knees. Drop your nonexercising arm by your side and bend the exercising arm at the elbow until your forearm is extending straight out from your body. Keep the bent elbow close to your side with your palm facing upward. Reach across with the nonexercising hand and place its palm under the hand on the exercising arm. Wrap the fingers of the nonexercising hand around the exercising hand between the base of the index finger and the thumb. Grasp gently. Without assisting, twist your exercising wrist so that the palm of your hand faces upward and outward and your thumb leads away from your body. You'll feel the stretch in your forearm. You may assist the end of the movement with your nonexercising hand.

Note: Right hand: 0° = 9:00. Left hand: 0° = 3:00.

Left Side

Range	Position on Clock	Degree of Range of Motion
Red Range Too tight	3:00–4:00	0°–30°
Yellow Range Normal	4:00–4:30	30°–45°
Green Range Elite athlete	4:30–5:00	45°–60°
Blue Range Hypermobile	5:00–6:00	60°–90°

Right Side

Range	Position on Clock	Degree of Range of Motion
Red Range Too tight	9:00–8:00	0°–30°
Yellow Range Normal	8:00–7:30	30°–45°
Green Range Elite athlete	7:30–7:00	45°–60°
Blue Range Hypermobile	7:00–6:00	60°–90°

Zone 4

40 Wrist Flexors—Palms Down

What You Stretch:	Muscles on the outsides of the forearms (flexor carpi radialis and flexor carpi ulnaris)
What You Contract:	Muscles on the insides of the forearms (extensor carpi radialis brevis and longus, and the extensor carpi ulnaris)
How Many Repetitions:	10 each side
How Long to Hold:	2 seconds

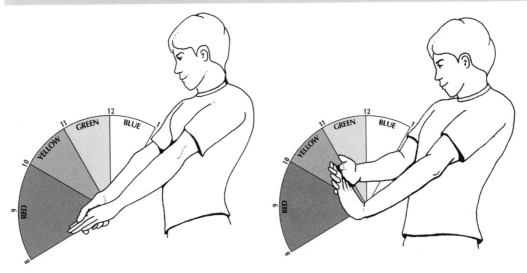

Note: This exercise also can be done while sitting on a chair.

Stand with your feet a few inches apart and slightly bend your knees. Hold the exercising arm straight in front of you and lock your elbow. "Cock" your hand up as if you were gesturing "Stop!" When the hand is in as upright a position as you can manage, the stretch happens. With the nonexercising hand, reach around the front of the fingers of the exercising hand and gently assist with a little pull back toward the body.

Note: 0° = 8:00.

Range	Position on Clock	Degree of Range of Motion
Red Range Too tight	8:00–10:00	0°–60°
Yellow Range Normal	10:00–11:00	60°–90°
Green Range Elite athlete	11:00–12:00	90°–120°
Blue Range Hypermobile	12:00–1:00	120°–150°

41 Wrist Flexors—Palms Up

What You Stretch:	Muscles on the outside of the forearms (flexor carpi radialis and flexor carpi ulnaris)
What You Contract:	Muscles on the inside of the forearms (extensor carpi radialis brevis and longus, and extensor carpi ulnaris)
How Many Repetitions:	10 each side
How Long to Hold:	2 seconds

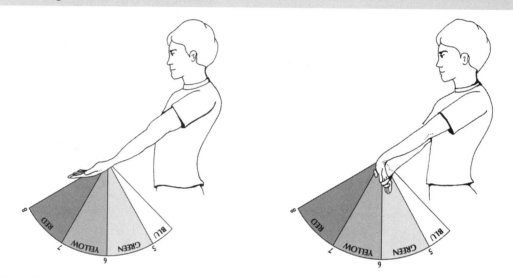

Note: This exercise also can be done while sitting on a chair.

Stand with your feet a few inches apart and your knees slightly bent. Hold the exercising arm straight in front of you and lock your elbow. Flip your hand over, palm up. Lead with your fingers to the floor until your palm is facing directly out from your body and your fingers are down. With the nonexercising hand, reach around to the front of the fingers of the exercising hand, and gently assist with a little pull back toward the body.

Note: 0° = 8:00.

Range	Position on Clock	Degree of Range of Motion
Red Range Too tight	8:00–7:00	0°–30°
Yellow Range Normal	7:00–6:00	30°–60°
Green Range Elite athlete	6:00–5:00	60°–90°
Blue Range Hypermobile	5:00–5:30	90°–105°

42 Wrist Extensors

What You Stretch:	Wrists and the outsides of the forearms (extensor carpi radialis longus, extensor carpi radialis brevis, and extensor carpi ulnaris)
What You Contract:	Wrists flexor muscles (flexor carpi radialis, and flexor carpi ulnaris)
How Many Repetitions:	10 each side
How Long to Hold:	2 seconds

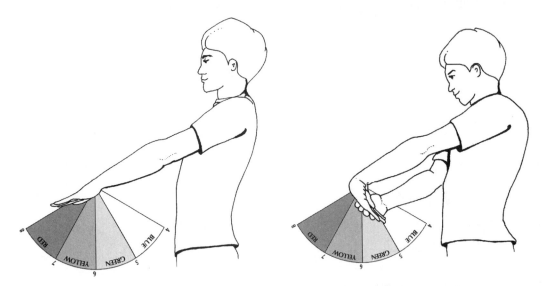

Note: This exercise also can be done while sitting on a chair.

Stand with your feet a few inches apart and your knees slightly bent. Hold the exercising arm straight in front of you and lock your elbow. Flip your hand over until your palm faces down. Extend your fingers. Bring your palm back toward your body as far as possible. With the nonexercising hand, reach around the top of the fingers of the exercising hand, and gently assist with a little pull back toward the body.

Note: 0° = 8:00.

Range	Position on Clock	Degree of Range of Motion
Red Range Too tight	8:00–7:00	0°–30°
Yellow Range Normal	7:00–6:00	30°–60°
Green Range Elite athlete	6:00–5:00	60°–90°
Blue Range Hypermobile	5:00–4:00	90°–120°

43   Finger Flexors

What You Stretch:	Fingers (flexor digitorum superficialis, flexor digitorum profundus and flexor digiti minimi)
What You Contract:	Fingers and the hand (extensor carpi radialis longus, extensor carpi radialis brevis, extensor carpi ulnaris, extensor digitorum, extensor indicis and extensor digiti minimi)
How Many Repetitions:	10 each side
How Long to Hold:	2 seconds

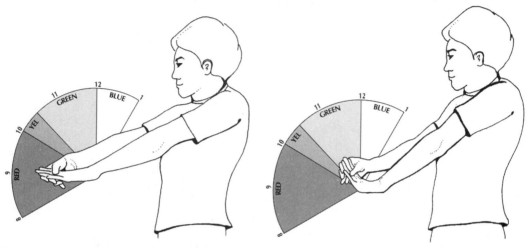

Note: This exercise also can be done while sitting on a chair.

Stand with your feet a few inches apart and your knees slightly bent. Hold the exercising arm straight in front of you and lock your elbow. "Cock" your hand upward as if you were gesturing "Stop!" With the nonexercising hand, reach around to the front of the exercising hand. Place your fingers against the fingertips of the stretching hand. Gently assist by pulling the straightened fingers back toward the body, keeping the wrist and palm still. A modification of this stretch is to stretch each finger individually. Remember: Do not allow the assisting hand to do all the work.

Note: 0° = 8:00.

Range	Position on Clock	Degree of Range of Motion
Red Range Too tight	8:00–11:00	0°–60°
Yellow Range Normal	10:00–10:30	60°–75°
Green Range Elite athlete	10:30–12:00	75°–90°
Blue Range Hypermobile	12:00–1:00	90°–120°

44 *Finger Extensors*

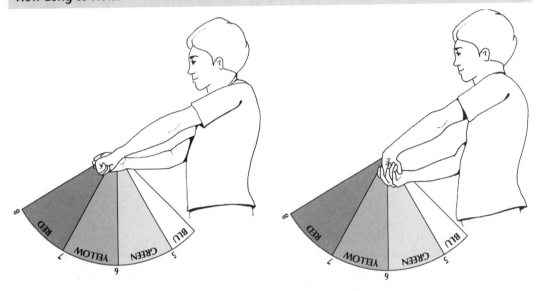

Note: This exercise also can be done while sitting on a chair.

Stand with your feet a few inches apart and your knees slightly bent. Hold the exercising arm straight in front of you and lock your elbow. Make a fist and bring it downward toward your body. With the nonexercising hand, reach around the front of your fist and grasp the knuckles. Gently assist by pulling your fist back toward your body.

Note: 0° = 8:00.

Range	Position on Clock	Degree of Range of Motion
Red Range Too tight	8:00–7:00	0°–30°
Yellow Range Normal	7:00–6:00	30°–60°
Green Range Elite athlete	6:00–5:00	60°–90°
Blue Range Hypermobile	5:00–5:30	90°–105°

Zone 4

45 *Finger Rotation*

What You Stretch:	Small finger muscles (extensor and flexors)
What You Contract:	Nothing. This is a passive stretch.
How Many Repetitions:	10 each side
How Long to Hold:	2 seconds

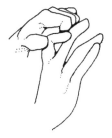 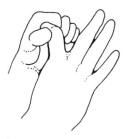 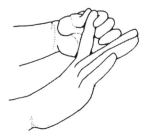

Note: This exercise also can be done while sitting on a chair.

This stretch is used to enhance the mobility of a joint that is locked up. Stand with your feet a few inches apart and your knees slightly bent. Gently grasp your exercising hand—palm up—with the opposite hand. Take each finger, one at a time, and rotate it to the left and then to the right. Repeat the same exercise with each finger bent at the large knuckle. The stretch should be a little deeper, because the bent finger acts like a lever, to help you stretch a little farther. Rotate each to the left and then to the right.

Zone 4

Range	Position on Clock	Degree of Range of Motion
Red Range Too tight		
Yellow Range Normal		
Green Range Elite athlete		
Blue Range Hypermobile		

What You Stretch:	Muscles and webbing between the fingers, the muscles between the thumb and the first finger (primarily the adductors including the adductor pollicis), and interossei palmaris
What You Contract:	Muscles and webbing between the fingers, the muscles between the thumb and the first finger (primarily the abductors including the abductor minimi digiti and the flexor brevis minimi digiti), and interossei dorsalis
How Many Repetitions:	10 each side
How Long to Hold:	2 seconds

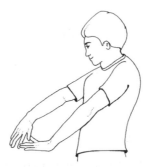

Note: This exercise can be done while sitting on a chair.

Stand with your feet a few inches apart and your knees slightly bent. Bring your exercising hand up in front of you by bending your elbow. Position your palm down and straighten your fingers. Extend the thumb out, away from the fingers. When you have extended it as far as you can, use your other hand to gently assist the "spread." Place your closed nonexercising hand between the exercising thumb and index finger and then slowly open it. Press each pair of exercising fingers apart. Repeat with the other hand.

This stretch releases tension between your fingers. You should be able to reach a 45° angle between each pair of fingers.

Zone 4

Range	Position on Clock	Degree of Range of Motion
Red Range Too tight		
Yellow Range Normal		
Green Range Elite athlete		
Blue Range Hypermobile		

Zone 5

Lower Legs, Ankles, and Feet

47 Soleus

What You Stretch:	Deep muscles in the back of the lower legs (soleus)
What You Contract:	Front of the lower legs (ankle–foot dorsal flexors, especially the tibialis anterior)
How Many Repetitions:	10 each side
How Long to Hold:	2 seconds

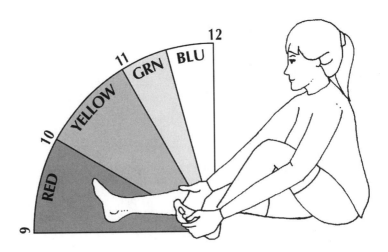

Sit with the nonexercising leg resting straight and flat in front of you. Bend the exercising leg at the knee, at a 90° angle. Place the foot flat on the surface of the floor or table. Reach down and grasp the bottom of your exercising foot with both hands. Keeping your heel on the surface and pivoting from your heel, raise the foot and bring it back toward your body as far as you can. Use your hands for a gentle assist at the end of the movement. If you are unable to reach your foot for this stretch, use your stretch rope. Make a loop and place it around your exercising foot, grasping the loose ends to stretch.

Zone 5

92

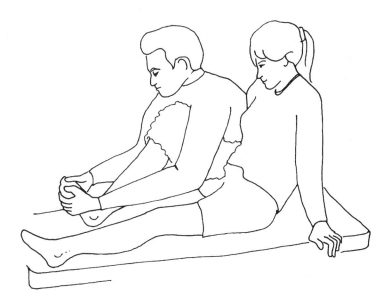

Assistant, sit beside your athlete. Let your athlete do all the work, but provide gentle assistance at the end. Grasp the forefoot of the exercising foot with both hands, and tuck the knee up under your arm. Apply a little pull for a 2-second hold.

Range	Position on Clock	Degree of Range of Motion
Red Range Too tight	9:00–10:00	0°–30°
Yellow Range Normal	10:00–11:00	30°–60°
Green Range Elite athlete	11:00–11:30	60°–75°
Blue Range Hypermobile	11:30–12:00	75°–90°

Zone 5

48　Achilles Tendon

What You Stretch:	The "cord" that attaches your heel to your lower leg (Achilles tendon)
What You Contract:	Front of the lower legs (ankle–foot dorsal flexors, especially the tibialis anterior)
How Many Repetitions:	10 each side
How Long to Hold:	2 seconds

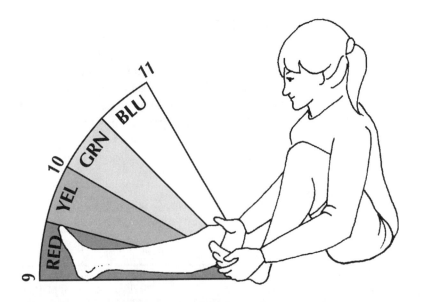

Sit with the nonexercising leg resting flat on the surface on which you are sitting. The exercising leg should be bent at the knee. Keep the foot flat, with the heel as close to the buttocks as possible. Grasp the bottom of the exercising foot with both hands. Raise the foot up, keeping the heel on the surface. A gentle assist with the hands may be used with this movement.

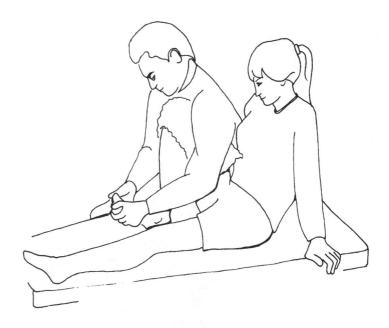

Assistant, sit beside your athlete. Let your athlete do all the work, but provide gentle assistance at the end. Grasp the forefoot of the exercising foot with both hands, and tuck the knee up under your arm. Apply a little pull for a 2-second hold.

Range	Position on Clock	Degree of Range of Motion
Red Range Too tight	9:00–9:30	0°–15°
Yellow Range Normal	9:30–10:00	15°–30°
Green Range Elite athlete	10:00–10:30	30°–45°
Blue Range Hypermobile	10:30–11:00	45°–60°

Zone 5

49 Gastrocnemius

What You Stretch:	Calf muscles (gastrocnemius)
What You Contract:	Muscles in fronts of the lower legs (ankle–foot dorsal flexors, especially the tibialis anterior)
How Many Repetitions:	10 each side
How Long to Hold:	2 seconds

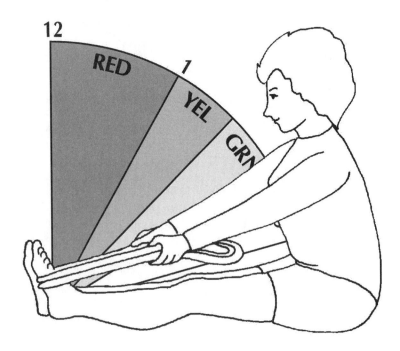

Sit with both legs straight out in front of you. To get the pressure off your back, you may want to relax your nonexercising leg by bending the knee and putting the sole of that foot flat on the surface on which you are sitting. Loop your rope around the foot of your exercising leg (still straight) and grasp each end of the rope in your hands. From your heel, flex your foot back toward your ankle, aiming your toes toward your knee. Use your rope for a gentle assist at the end of this movement. Remember to keep your knee locked and upper body still. For an advanced stretch, you may bend forward at your hips and lean your upper body closer to your locked knee.

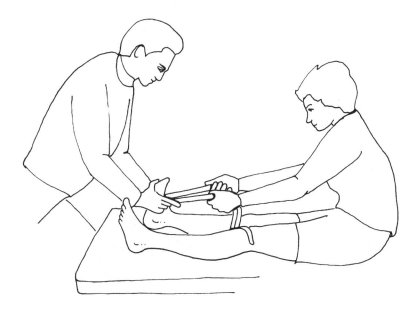

Assistant, let your athlete use the rope and do all the work, but provide gentle assistance at the end. Wrap both hands around the ball of the exercising foot. Apply a little push for a 2-second hold. As the joint opens up, it will be possible for your athlete to bend forward at the hips with the back straight, for a deeper stretch. Please remind him or her to keep that knee locked.

Range	Position on Clock	Degree of Range of Motion
Red Range Too tight	12:00–1:00	0°–30°
Yellow Range Normal	1:00–1:30	30°–45°
Green Range Elite athlete	1:30–2:00	45°–60°
Blue Range Hypermobile	2:00–2:30	60°–75°

Zone 5

50 *Tibialis Anterior*

What You Stretch:	Muscles in the fronts of the lower legs (ankle–foot dorsal flexors, especially the tibialis anterior and extensor digitorum muscles)
What You Contract:	Muscles in the backs of the lower legs (plantaris, soleus, gastrocnemius, and the flexor digitorum)
How Many Repetitions:	10 each side
How Long to Hold:	2 seconds

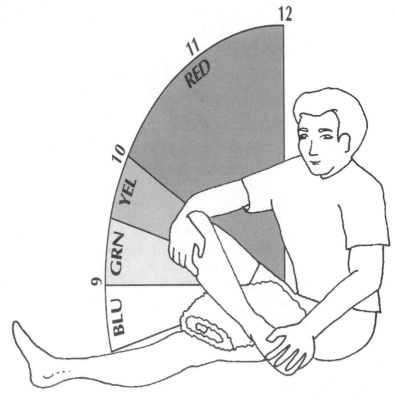

Note: You may want to use a folded towel on the top of your thigh, under the ankle of your exercising leg.

Sit with both legs straight in front of you, resting flat on the surface on which you are sitting. Bring the foot of the exercising leg up and place it on top of the thigh—just above the knee—of the nonexercising leg. Reach straight down and grasp the exercising forefoot with your hand, on the side of the nonexercising leg. Use the other hand to apply gentle pressure on the inside of the knee of the exercising leg, to stabilize it. Point (flex) your exercising foot. You may use your hand for a gentle assist at the end of your stretch. To modify this stretch, pull up slightly at the end of the movement, to stretch the tibialis posterior.

Zone 5

When Two Heads Are Better Than One . . .

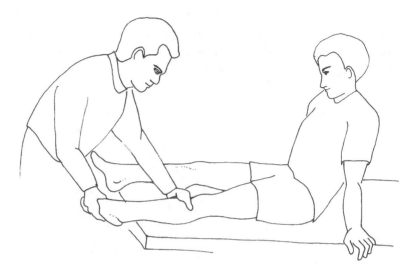

Note: When you're visualizing your clockface, start with your
foot perpendicular to your lower leg. The clock is beside
your foot. Your toes are at 12:00.

Assistant, let your athlete do all the work, but provide
gentle assistance at the end. Place one hand on the shin to stabilize, and one hand on the top of the forefoot. Apply a little
push for a 2-second hold. A modification of this stretch is to
turn the foot inward as you push.

Note: 0° = 12:00.

Range	Position on Clock	Degree of Range of Motion
Red Range Too tight	12:00–10:00	0°–60°
Yellow Range Normal	10:00–9:30	60°–75°
Green Range Elite athlete	9:30–9:00	75°–90°
Blue Range Hypermobile	9:00–8:30	90°–105°

Zone 5

51 Ankle Evertors

What You Stretch:	Muscles of the outside of the feet and lower legs (peroneus longus, peroneus brevis, peroneus tertius, and extensor digitorum longus)
What You Contract:	Inside of the feet and ankles (tibialis posterior and tibialis anterior)
How Many Repetitions:	10 each side
How Long to Hold:	2 seconds

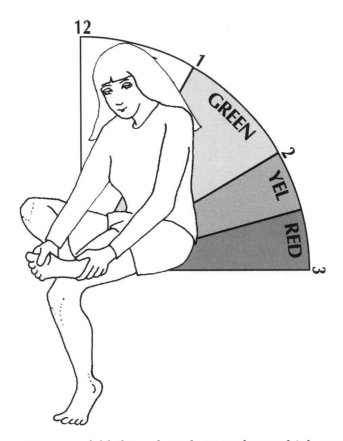

Note: You may want to use a folded towel on the top of your thigh, under the ankle of your exercising leg.

Sit with both legs resting straight in front of you, flat on the surface on which you are sitting. Bring the foot of the exercising leg up and place it on top of the thigh—just above the knee—of the nonexercising leg. Reach straight down and grasp your exercising forefoot with your hands, on the side of the nonexercising leg. From the ankle, rotate your foot inward, pointing the sole of that foot up. You may use your hand for a gentle assist at the end of your stretch.

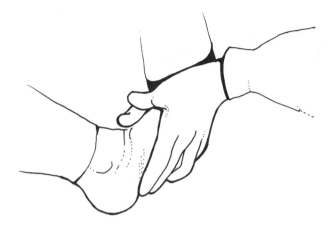

Assistant, sit beside your athlete. Let your athlete do all the work, but provide gentle assistance at the end. Wrap both hands around the midfoot. Apply a little rotation inward for a 2-second hold.

Left Side

Range	Position on Clock	Degree of Range of Motion
Red Range Too tight	9:00–9:30	0°–15°
Yellow Range Normal	9:30–10:00	15°–30°
Green Range Elite athlete	10:00–11:00	30°–60°
Blue Range Hypermobile	11:00–12:00	60°–90°

Right Side

Range	Position on Clock	Degree of Range of Motion
Red Range Too tight	3:00–2:30	0°–15°
Yellow Range Normal	2:30–2:00	15°–30°
Green Range Elite athlete	2:00–1:00	30°–60°
Blue Range Hypermobile	1:00–12:00	60°–90°

Zone 5

52 Ankle Invertors

What You Stretch: Muscles of the ankles (tibialis posterior and tibialis anterior)

What You Contract: Ankles (peroneus longus, peroneus brevis, peroneus tertius, and extensor digitorum longus)

How Many Repetitions: 10 each side

How Long to Hold: 2 seconds

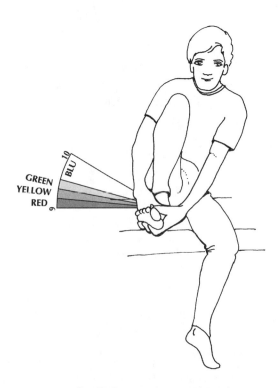

Sit in a chair or on the edge of a table. Bring the foot of the exercising leg up and place it on the surface in front of your buttock. Reach straight down and grasp the exercising forefoot with your hand, on the side of the nonexercising leg. Use the other hand to apply gentle pressure on the inside of the knee of the exercising leg, to stabilize it. From the ankle, rotate your foot outward from the middle of your body. You may use your hand for a gentle assist at the end of your stretch.

102

When Two Heads Are Better Than One . . .

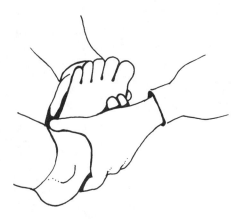

Assistant, sit beside your athlete. Let your athlete do all the work, but provide gentle assistance at the end. Wrap both hands around the midfoot. Apply a little rotation outward for a 2-second hold.

Left Side

Range	Position on Clock	Degree of Range of Motion
Red Range Too tight	3:00–2:50	0°–5°
Yellow Range Normal	2:50–2:40	5°–10°
Green Range Elite athlete	2:40–2:30	10°–15°
Blue Range Hypermobile	2:30–2:00	15°–30°

Right Side

Range	Position on Clock	Degree of Range of Motion
Red Range Too tight	9:00–9:10	0°–5°
Yellow Range Normal	9:10–9:20	5°–10°
Green Range Elite athlete	9:20–9:30	10°–15°
Blue Range Hypermobile	9:30–10:00	15°–30°

Zone 5

53 Foot Pronators

What You Stretch:	The insertions of the muscles in your feet that rotate to the outside (peroneus longus, peroneus brevis, peroneus tertius, and extensor digitorum longus)
What You Contract:	The insertions of the muscles in your feet that rotate to the inside (gastrocnemius, soleus, flexor hallucis longus, flexor digitorum longus, tibialis anterior, and tibialis posterior)
How Many Repetitions:	10 each side
How Long to Hold:	2 seconds

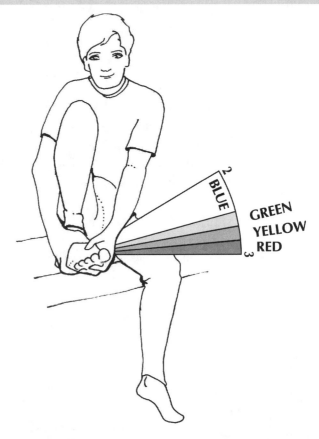

Sit on a chair or on the edge of a table. Let your lower legs dangle over the side, hanging loosely from your knees. Bring the foot of the exercising leg up to the surface on which you are sitting. Stabilize your position by grasping your heel with the hand from the opposite side. Grasp the exercising forefoot at the base of the toes, with your arm against the inside of your leg. Turn your forefoot in and up. Gently assist with your hand at the end of the movement.

When Two Heads Are Better Than One . . .

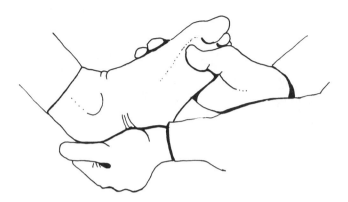

Assistant, sit beside your athlete. Let your athlete do all the work, but provide gentle assistance at the end. Hold the heel in the palm of one hand, and hold the forefoot with the other. Apply a little rotation inward for a 2-second hold.

Left Side

Range	Position on Clock	Degree of Range of Motion
Red Range Too tight	9:00–9:10	0°–5°
Yellow Range Normal	9:10–9:20	5°–10°
Green Range Elite athlete	9:20–9:30	10°–15°
Blue Range Hypermobile	9:30–9:40	15°–20°

Right Side

Range	Position on Clock	Degree of Range of Motion
Red Range Too tight	3:00–2:50	0°–5°
Yellow Range Normal	2:50–2:40	5°–10°
Green Range Elite athlete	2:40–2:30	10°–15°
Blue Range Hypermobile	2:30–2:20	15°–20°

Zone 5

54 Foot Supinators

What You Stretch:	The attachments of the muscles in your feet that rotate to the inside (gastrocnemius, soleus, flexor hallucis longus, flexor digitorum longus, tibialis anterior, and tibialis posterior)
What You Contract:	The attachments of the muscles in your feet that rotate to the outside (peroneus longus, peroneus brevis, peroneus tertius, and extensor digitorum longus)
How Many Repetitions:	10 each side
How Long to Hold:	2 seconds

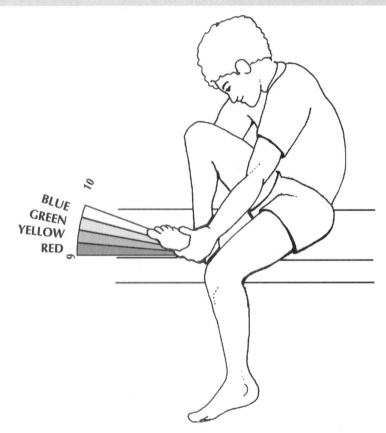

BLUE
GREEN
YELLOW
RED

Sit on a chair or on the edge of a table. Let your lower legs dangle over the side, hanging loosely from your knees. Bring the foot of the exercising leg up to the surface on which you are sitting. Stabilize your position by grasping your heel with the hand from the opposite side. Grasp the exercising forefoot at the base of the toes, with your arm against the outside of your leg. Turn your forefoot out and up. Gently assist with your hand at the end of the movement.

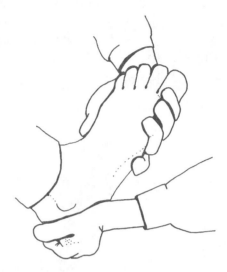

Assistant, sit beside your athlete. Let your athlete do all the work, but provide gentle assistance at the end. Hold the heel in the palm of one hand, and hold the forefoot with the other. Apply a little rotation outward for a 2-second hold.

Left Side

Range	Position on Clock	Degree of Range of Motion
Red Range Too tight	3:00–2:50	0°–5°
Yellow Range Normal	2:50–2:40	5°–10°
Green Range Elite athlete	2:40–2:30	10°–15°
Blue Range Hypermobile	2:30–2:20	15°–20°

Right Side

Range	Position on Clock	Degree of Range of Motion
Red Range Too tight	9:00–9:10	0°–5°
Yellow Range Normal	9:10–9:20	5°–10°
Green Range Elite athlete	9:20–9:30	10°–15°
Blue Range Hypermobile	9:30–9:40	15°–20°

Zone 5

55 Metatarsal Arch

What You Stretch:	Muscles on the bottom of your feet, just behind the balls of your feet (transverse fibers of the forefoot)
What You Contract:	Muscles that flex your toes (including the flexor digitorum brevis longus and flexor hallucis longus)
How Many Repetitions:	10 each side
How Long to Hold:	2 seconds

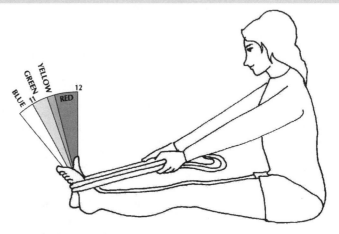

Sit with both legs resting straight out in front of you. To get the pressure off your back, you may want to relax your nonexercising leg by bending the knee and putting the sole of that foot flat on the surface on which you are sitting. Loop your rope around the foot of your exercising leg (still straight), placing the loop just beneath the ball of your foot. Grasp each end of the rope in your hands.

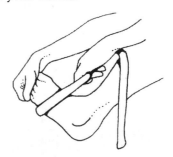

You can also perform this stretch seated, with your knee bent at a 90° angle. From your heel, flex your foot back toward your ankle, aiming your toes toward your knee. Hold that position with your rope and curl your toes tightly down. Remember to keep your knee locked and your upper body still. Grasp your toes and press gently down.

When Two Heads Are Better Than One . . .

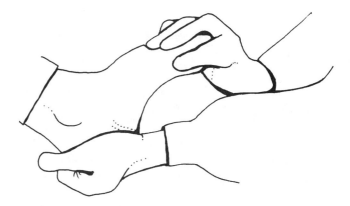

Assistant, sit beside your athlete. Let your athlete do all the work, but provide gentle assistance at the end. Bend and flex the toes (back and forth) for a 2-second hold. You can manipulate the toes individually or all together.

Range	Position on Clock	Degree of Range of Motion
Red Range Too tight	12:00–12:30	0°–15°
Yellow Range Normal	12:30–12:40	15°–20°
Green Range Elite athlete	12:40–1:00	20°–30°
Blue Range Hypermobile	1:00–1:20	30°–40°

56   Toe Extensors

What You Stretch:	Muscles on the top of the toes that help the toes to curl up (extensor hallucis longus and brevis)
What You Contract:	Muscles on the bottom of the toes that help the toes to curl down (flexor hallucis longus and brevis)
How Many Repetitions:	10 each side
How Long to Hold:	2 seconds

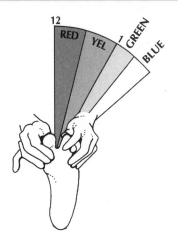

Sit on a flat surface with both legs resting straight in front of you. Bend the exercising leg at the knee at a 90° angle, and place the foot flat on the surface. Reach down and grasp the bottom of your exercising foot with both hands. Keeping your heel on the surface and pivoting from your heel, raise your foot and curl your toes tightly down toward the surface. Use your hand to press against the top of your toes and assist them as they move down and back. As a modification of this stretch, you can flex each toe individually

When Two Heads Are Better Than One . . .

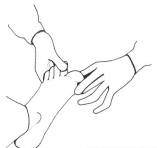

Assistant, sit beside your athlete. Let your athlete do all the work, but provide gentle assistance at the end. Flex the toes downward for a 2-second hold. You can flex the toes individually or all together.

Range	Position on Clock	Degree of Range of Motion
Red Range Too tight	12:00–12:30	0°–15°
Yellow Range Normal	12:30–1:00	15°–30°
Green Range Elite athlete	1:00–1:20	30°–40°
Blue Range Hypermobile	1:20–1:30	40°–60°

57   Toe Flexors

What You Stretch:	Muscles on the bottom of the toes that help the toes to curl down (flexor hallucis longus and brevis)
What You Contract:	Muscles on the top of the toes that help the toes to curl up (extensor hallucis longus and brevis)
How Many Repetitions:	10 each side
How Long to Hold:	2 seconds

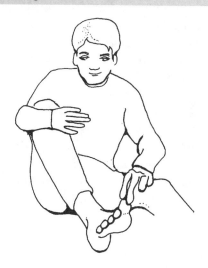

Sit on a flat surface with both legs resting straight in front of you. Bend the exercising leg at the knee, at a 90° angle, and place the foot flat on the surface. Reach down and grasp the bottom of your exercising foot with both hands. Keeping your heel on the surface and pivoting from your heel, raise your foot and bring your toes back toward your body. Use your hand to press against the bottom of your toes and assist them as they hyperextend toward your body. As a modification of this stretch, you can assist each toe individually.

When Two Heads Are Better Than One . . .

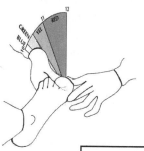

Assistant, sit beside your athlete. Let your athlete do all the work, but provide gentle assistance at the end. Extend the toes upward for a 2-second hold. You can extend the toes individually or all together.

Range	Position on Clock	Degree of Range of Motion
Red Range Too tight	12:00–11:00	0°–30°
Yellow Range Normal	11:00–10:30	30°–45°
Green Range Elite athlete	10:30–10:20	45°–55°
Blue Range Hypermobile	10:20–10:00	55°–60°

Zone 5

111

58   Big Toe Adductor

What You Stretch:	Big toes (adductor hallucis)
What You Contract:	Big toes (abductor hallucis)
How Many Repetitions:	10 each toe
How Long to Hold:	2 seconds

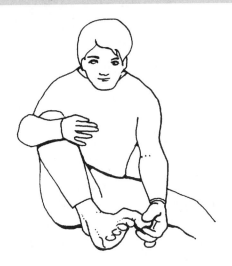

Sit on a flat surface with both legs resting straight in front of you. Bend the exercising leg at the knee, at a 90° angle, and place the foot flat on the surface. Reach down and grasp the bottom of your exercising foot with both hands. Keeping your heel on the surface and pivoting from your heel, raise your foot slightly. Move your big toe away from your other toes—to the outside. Use your fingers to assist gently at the end of the movement. (If your toe is too weak to move, your toe will position itself to the inside—a condition called hallux valgus—and put you at risk for a bunion.)

When Two Heads Are Better Than One . . .

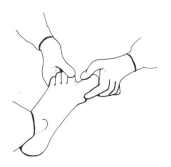

Assistant, sit beside your athlete. Let your athlete do all the work, but provide gentle assistance at the end. Hold the exercising forefoot in one hand and use the fingers of the other hand to move the big toe away from the other toes for a 2-second hold.

Range	Position on Clock	Degree of Range of Motion
Red Range Too tight		
Yellow Range Normal		
Green Range Elite athlete		
Blue Range Hypermobile		

59 Toe Webbing

What You Stretch:	Toes (deep transverse metatarsal ligaments, extensor digitorum longus tendons, and flexor digitorum tendons)
What You Contract:	Toes (adductors and abductors)
How Many Repetitions:	10 each toe
How Long to Hold:	2 seconds

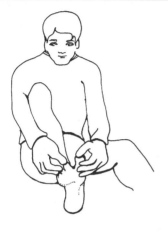

Sit on a flat surface with both legs resting straight in front of you. Bend the exercising leg at the knee, at a 90° angle, and place the foot flat on the surface. Keeping your heel on the surface and pivoting from your heel, raise your foot slightly. Spread your toes. Use your fingers to assist gently at the end of the movement by widening the spaces between the toes, one pair at a time.

When Two Heads Are Better Than One . . .

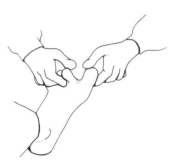

Assistant, sit beside your athlete. Let your athlete do all the work, but provide gentle assistance at the end. Spread the toes, one pair at a time, for a 2-second hold.

There is no specific range of motion for the toes. Generally, you should be able to reach a 45° spread between each pair.

Range	Position on Clock	Degree of Range of Motion
Red Range Too tight		
Yellow Range Normal		
Green Range Elite athlete		
Blue Range Hypermobile		

Zone 5

Part II
Selecting Your Active-Isolated Stretches

OK, Athlete! It's time to plan your strategy. To decide which stretches you need in your program, identify all the sports and occupational activities that you do now or that you *know* you will be doing on a regular basis. If you live in Kansas and have no vacation coming, you can skip Wind Surfing.

Match your list against the index on pages xi–xii at the front of the book. Those are the sections that will be of special interest to you now. If you decide to train for an additional sport, or your activities change with the seasons, you have here all the information you need to get in shape for new activities you may add to your list.

At the start of the discussion of each activity, we note the zones of the body you will need for performance of the activity and the numbers of the stretches that you should make part of your program. You'll find some overlap if you engage in more than one sport. Block out all the stretches required for your particular activities. Then mesh them so that your stretching program is smoothly coordinated to prepare you for whatever activities are included in your daily or weekly schedule.

For every sport and occupational activity, we give you a "Coaches' Notes" section—professional advice and information that will enhance any program that you are planning.

Read through all of the offerings in the Sports and Occupational Activities sections of this part of the book. You will gain appreciation for some sports you do not perform. And you may find some that are worth looking into. Almost everyone earmarks several topics that are of personal interest!

Have copies of your Personal Active-Isolated Stretching Program form handy (see the "Forms to Photocopy" at the back of the book), and let's get started!

Sports

Aerobics/Aerobic Dancing

Stretches:	Upper Legs, Hips, and Trunk	1–17
	Shoulders	18–27
	Neck	28–34
	Arms, Elbows, Wrists, and Hands	35–46
	Lower Legs, Ankles, and Feet	47–59

Coaches' Notes

Aerobics offers a terrific cardiovascular workout, but if not done properly, can result in overuse: injuries of the lower back, hips, legs, ankles and feet; strains, tendinitis, and stress fractures. Using ankle weights, handheld dumbbells, or steps tends to increase the possibility of injury. The fitness industry, recognizing the risks, has developed low-impact or no-impact programs. Indeed, we have seen aerobics classes conducted in chest-deep water: "aquacise."

Look for classes held on floors that yield when you step down. Working out for hours every day on a concrete floor is asking for trouble. Wearing high-tech shoes specifically designed for aerobic dance may give you some support and cushioning, and assist in maintaining proper foot position, but shoes can't compensate entirely for a surface that is too hard. Carpeting doesn't help. The shock absorption system in the foot is remarkable, but repeated hammering will translate forces right up the leg to the hips and back. At first, you might feel only sore feet and tired legs. Eventually, without a rest from the relentless pounding, something may fatigue, then strain, then break.

Protect yourself from injury by preparing for every class with an Active-Isolated Stretching warm-up. Be alert for unfamiliar moves that put your body into new positions. Another risk is impact resulting in a traumatic injury. For example, if you boot-scoot left when the rest of the people in line boot-scoot right, the result will be an ugly pileup, with cuts and bruises. You might also injure yourself by falling off a step platform or by stepping down badly during a maneuver. It's best to take classes commensurate with your level of ability until you feel confident and ready to advance. We suggest that you study with a certified, experienced aerobics instructor. Ask to see credentials, interview the instructor before you sign up for the class, and talk to some other students. We want you to have fun, but we also want you to be safe and in competent, qualified hands!

We use aerobic dancing as a complement to training regimens, but we are aware that, for some dancers, the aerobics programs are the primary activities. If you are one of these people, we advise you to consider supplementing your training with strength and flexibility workouts.

Drink plenty of fluids before and after your workout. Warm up and cool down without fail. Invest in shoes specifically designed for aerobic dancing. And go out and have a ball!

Baseball/Softball

Stretches:		
	Upper Legs, Hips, and Trunk	1–17
	Shoulders	18–27
	Neck	28–34
	Arms, Elbows, Wrists, and Hands	35–46
	Lower Legs, Ankles, and Feet	47–59

Coaches' Notes

Baseball is considered to be a safe noncontact sport that requires a minimum of protective equipment. In fact, its risk of injury is ranked last among competitive sports. Ironically, however, baseball ranks second—right behind football—in *total number* of injuries. This confusing statistic originates from the large number of participants, from children to seniors. This popular sport is enjoyed by many casual and dedicated players, some of whom get injured.

When we consider the typical baseball injuries, we know that many of them are caused by relative inactivity followed by explosive movement. Picture yourself standing alone at an outfield position. A fly ball pops your way, and you instantly scramble at top speed. Or, after five innings of sitting on the bench in the dugout, you're called to pinch-hit, and you bolt up to bat. Your body sometimes has difficulty adjusting from rest to sudden activity. We encourage you to keep moving. Use every minute to stay warmed up with stretching, getting ready for your heroic moment.

Individual dynamics of baseball are throwing, sprinting, hitting, sliding, catching, and fielding.

Throwing is a total body activity that requires a delicate balance between mobility and stability. It may look like an action of your arm and shoulder, but your whole body, starting with your legs and trunk, gets into the act—and the acts gets even trickier if you are throwing while running or jumping. Any time a baseball or softball player doubts our assertion that the lower body is heavily involved in throwing or pitching, we strap him or her into a chair and then challenge the player to throw the ball a tenth of the distance he or she is used to throwing it. We gain a believer every time. From stance, a thrower has wind-up, cocking, acceleration, and deceleration (followed by elation and jubilation—if the ball goes where intended).

121

Sprinting in baseball requires thrust from the hip and trunk, agility from the foot and ankle, and power from the shoulders and pumping arms. Notice that we are not talking about "running." You seldom run in baseball; you rarely have that luxury of time. You need to get where you're going in an instant. You'll go from a standing or crouched position into a sprint down the baseline or to make a play. You have to stop quickly, and then initiate another move such as throwing, catching, tagging, or sliding. The sequence takes great skill and care.

In hitting, the primary stress point is your knee. Surprised? We see dislocated kneecaps from sudden twisting and pivoting around a planted foot. Shoe spikes hold the ground well—too well, in some instances. Also, you need to be careful of your wrists and trunk.

Sliding is responsible for a large portion of baseball injuries. When you slide, keep your face off the bases and home plate, the ground, and the shoes (and spikes) of other players. Impact always carries a risk of injuring yourself and someone else. Whether you prefer a head-first or a feet-first slide, you are converting a vertical stance into a horizontal position against a surface and at high speed. Sliding requires flexibility and strength to avoid damaging ankles, feet, hips, trunk, wrists, fingers—and face.

A team's catcher just might play the most physically demanding position: squatting and standing, catching and throwing, chasing balls, and avoiding collisions with balls, bats, base runners, and misplaced umpires. Think of the stress on your knees (squatting), shoulder (throwing), and hands (impact from ball).

In fielding, we see explosive bursts of muscle activity from a fixed position. Success requires coordination, flexibility, sudden sprinting, and changing direction. You can avoid injury by maintaining strength and flexibility, with emphasis on hip and trunk, shoulder, forearm, wrist, and finger flexors.

Basketball

Stretches:	Upper Legs, Hips, and Trunk	1–17
	Shoulders	18–27
	Neck	28–34
	Arms, Elbows, Wrists, and Hands	35–46
	Lower Legs, Ankles, and Feet	47–59

Coaches' Notes

Basketball, from our perspective, is a collision sport. Most injuries occur when a player meets head-on with another player, a spectator, the backboard, the floor, and so on. Repetitive performance of complex and ballistic movements characterizes the sport: running, jumping, rapidly changing direction, rotating, and throwing. Unfortunately, the very nature of these movements, which sharpens up an athlete's body, also puts a player at risk of physical injury, particularly to tendons, ligaments, and muscles that stabilize joints. Landing from a layup, for example, produces forces seven times your body weight; a jump shot produces forces five times your body weight. And no one has yet approved a basketball court floor that is soft enough to assist you in absorbing those forces when you come down.

In descending order of their stress demands, your body's most injury-prone points are knee, ankle, lower back, shin, hip, shoulder, neck, wrist, foot, groin, and fingers. Among basketball players, we see some overuse injuries in these areas, so be conscientious about proper stretching and conditioning.

Please, be *very* selective in purchasing your shoes. Specifically designed basketball shoes that have a little cushioning can compensate slightly for a hard floor. Beware of shoes that are too soft, however. You do need support for all the work you're about to do. Additionally, basketball shoes are "high-topped" with ankle support. Do not make the mistake of playing in running shoes. Their soles are designed to keep you moving forward and are not very good for pivoting. When you play to win, you need every advantage you can get—beginning with the right shoes.

Bodybuilding

Stretches:	Upper Legs, Hips, and Trunk	1–17
	Shoulders	18–27
	Arms, Elbows, Wrists, and Hands	35–46
	Lower Legs, Ankles, and Feet	47–59

Coaches' Notes

It is very distressing to look at a bodybuilder and realize that he or she is not fit. The contradiction occurs frequently. In our definition, "fitness" is comprised of health, strength, cardiovascular fitness (endurance), and flexibility. The great irony of being a bodybuilder is that you may have only ONE of those components: strength. You look great, but you may be in lousy shape. To excel in your sport, your goal should be to put all the fitness pieces in place. As an added benefit, you'll last longer, both in the gym and in your life.

In this sport, flexibility is a vital element of both competition and training. More elastic muscles have more room to grow, and this means more mass, symmetry, and definition. Additionally, the more flexible a muscle is, the shorter the recovery time after intense lifting. You'll be able to lift more weight for longer periods of time. The principle is fairly easy to understand. When you lift, a muscle strains, sustaining a series of micro-tears. Its subsequent recovery from this trauma is what makes the muscle stronger, adapting it to the increasing weight loads you impose on it. When a muscle is flexible and elastic, it is able to more quickly flush out the metabolic wastes resulting from the tears suffered during the lift. Quicker flushing means quicker recovery. And quicker recovery means accelerating the tear-down/build-up cycle that develops a muscle.

Sculpted, developed muscles are "what it's all about" on the bodybuilding circuit. Muscles that are elongated from origin to insertion (or proximal to distal attachment) show off the muscle striations and "cuts." You'll look great in competition on a stage under the lights. And the benefits of flexibility don't stop here. The more flexibility you have, the more varied, difficult, and exciting you can make the choreography in your routine.

A special word of caution to female bodybuilders. Allowing your body fat content to drop below 16 percent in order to achieve a "cut" look may cause your estrogen levels to diminish, possibly resulting in your losing estrogen's cardioprotective properties, developing amenorrhea, and running an increased risk of osteoporosis. Every woman is different, so you and your physician will want to monitor your body carefully.

Bowling

Stretches:		
Upper Legs, Hips, and Trunk	1–17	
Shoulders	18–27	
Arms, Elbows, Wrists, and Hands	35–46	

Coaches' Notes

You have two missions in bowling: (1) get into position on the line and (2) release the ball so that it scorches down the lane and shatters all the pins into splinters. Strong legs allow you to control your approach and to get into and hold your perfect release position. Your hip flexors and buttocks assist you in propelling the ball straight forward. Your back, shoulders, arms, wrists, and hands have quite an interesting challenge. They have to be powerful enough to lift and thrust the ball, but still able to give you the delicate finesse you'll need to fine-tune your aim and put your special spin on the ball. It's an unusual combination; it requires training, conditioning, and practice.

Here's an inside pointer into scoping out the weakness of your competition. We all know that it is fashionable to wear a wrist guard from the elbow to the palm of the hand while bowling. It makes a bowler look ferocious. You are supposed to take one look at a wrist guard on an opponent's arm and think, "This bowler is SERIOUS—bowls SO much that the hand needs to be shored up. I am in deep trouble here." Think again. If a bowler is wearing a wrist guard, he or she is weak and getting weaker all the time. It is much more fashionable and ferocious to hoist your ball into the air with a wrist and hand so strong and flexible that you don't need to be braced. Besides, you'll catch everyone off guard, giving yourself a competitive advantage. Strength and flexibility are crucial to a perfect 300.

Boxing

Stretches:	Upper Legs, Hips, and Trunk	1–17
	Shoulders	18–27
	Neck	28–34
	Arm and Wrist	35–41
	Ankle and Foot	41–59

Coaches' Notes

We aren't crazy about any sport where the winner is declared only after he or she has pounded another human being into submission, but we are crazy about the no-frills training approach to boxing. We hope you'll emphasize the training and leave the pounding to the professionals. If you do decide to go into a ring with an opponent, we are trusting you to (1) wear all the protective gear you can find (especially for your head, face, and eyes, where most injuries in boxing are incurred), (2) box under the supervision of a trained professional coach, and (3) spar with a partner of equal ability who understands that these rounds are for fun. Our clients who train to box swear that they get great workouts and are guaranteed dramatic stress reduction. One said, "It's either the punching bag or my boss. The choice is fairly easy." We understand.

But let's concentrate on the training components and their contributions to your fitness program. Distance running and cycling will give you cardiovascular endurance. Wind sprints will give you fast-twitch muscle fiber conditioning and increased anaerobic capacity. Jumping rope will increase your endurance, leg speed, and coordination. Speed bag is great for increasing hand speed, eye–hand coordination, and reflex action. Heavy bag enhances your punching power, general conditioning, and stamina. Strength training builds muscle;

you should know that most boxers train with light, free weights. Stretching and flexibility will warm up your body for the workout and help you maximize your performance on every level. Sparring develops eye-hand coordination and allows you to "put it all together"—provided your opponent is not bent on taking you all apart.

Let us say it again. The training for boxing is stellar and we support it. Boxing in the ring is dangerous and should be left to the professionals.

Canoeing

Stretches:	Upper Legs, Hips, and Trunk	1–17
	Shoulders	18–27
	Arms, Elbows, Wrists, and Hands	35–46

Coaches' Notes

When we think of canoeing, we think *Relaxation*. Rhythmic stroking of the paddle. Gliding over sparkling water. A sunny day. A guy with a ukelele. A gal with a parasol. The whole scene is so idyllic, and SO deceptive. The truth is that canoeing is an endurance sport and a highly competitive Olympic event that requires power, stamina, balance, and skill. Believe us, the ukelele and parasol are optional props. Romance notwithstanding, canoeing engages your whole body in performance. There are critical musculoskeletal factors in being able to do it well.

You'll be using your arm flexors—biceps and forearm flexors and extensors—to raise the paddle out of the water and begin the motion of bringing it forward. When you bring it to the start of a stroke and lower your arm, your chest, back of the upper arm (triceps), sides of the upper back (lats), upper back muscles (teres major), and muscles under the shoulder blades (subscapularis) all contribute to controlling your movement.

Your trunk allows you to do the paddling motion. You use your abdominals when your trunk flexes forward as the paddle enters the water. Your back (erector spinae) supports your arms as you pull the paddle through the water and return it to position. Your back essentially powers your stroke. Even though you are seated, you use your legs in the pulling phase of paddling. You'll notice increased tension in your hips and knees as you brace yourself in the seat. You brace by extending and locking your knees and ankles during the pulling phase. The brace also gives you balance.

Remember that paddling is a repetitive motion and you run the risk of "overuse syndrome" in your hands, wrists, and arms. You may develop nerve impingements, pain, numbness, and severe fatigue. If you are strong and flexible, if you change positions from time to time, and if you stay relaxed, you minimize the risk. Also, you'll have more fun!

Cricket

Coaches' Notes

Cricket, like many team sports, is a wonderful way to stay fit while you enjoy the added benefit of the company of your friends and teammates. Also, playing a team sport infuses your training program with incentives and motivations. You want to do your best to help your buddies win, so you put in extra time and effort off the playing field. And, just when you think you can't get any better, you step out onto the cricket field, get a jolt of that indescribable team spirit and a few assists, and suddenly are able to drive your personal performance beyond your wildest expectations. You know. You've had those days. They're why you play cricket.

Cricket, at first glance, is a fairly low-injury game played by incredibly civilized gentlemen and gentlewomen wearing pressed white uniforms and abiding by polite rules that have governed the game since antiquity. We are not deceived. We know it's low-injury because of the protective gear you wear: a helmet fitted with a shatterproof face visor, a high-impact-resistant chest protector, forearm guard, gloves, genital protector, thigh pads, and shin pads. And just what is being protected against? A little 5.5-ounce ball rocketing right at you at a scorching *90* miles per hour.

Getting nailed with the ball is not your only concern; padding, coordination, lightning reflexes, and a dead-eye bowler will take care of that peril. You need to anticipate and prepare for a series of other potential problems, the solutions to which are fully in your control. Because your back foot must remain on the ground when you bat, your Achilles tendon could suffer irritation; you run the risk of rupture. Your knee, if you are the wicket keeper, may strain and fatigue from squatting for long periods of time. Your back, when bowling or batting, needs to be strong and flexible in order to avoid straining. Wrists and hands (especially if you are the wicket keeper) are subjected to continuous microtrauma from throwing and catching. And your shoulder requires particular attention. The most commonly injured joint in cricket, it is most often damaged in throwing. Without flexibility and a generous joint range of motion, you will inevitably put additional stress on your shoulder rotators (that group of muscles called collectively "the rotator cuff"). A common result of this mistake is impingement—muscles tighten around a nerve, causing numbing, weakening, loss of motor response, and pain.

You'll play better and enjoy your game more if you are in shape—strong and flexible. And your teammates certainly will appreciate the results of your efforts.

Cross-Country Skiing

Stretches:	Upper Legs, Hips, and Trunk	1–17
	Shoulders	18–27
	Lower Legs, Ankles, and Feet	47–59

Coaches' Notes

Skis have been used for over 4,500 years in Scandinavia. Until the popularity and availability of the snowmobile, cross-country skiing was an important means of transportation through the snowy back country. Interestingly, this ancient sport is changing rapidly today, due to emerging technologies in materials. The old wooden skis provided limited glide capacity. Today's Fiberglas™ and graphite skis are smoother and slicker on the surface of snow. Increased glide means that the skier has to be stronger to control the action and take advantage of it to cover greater distances more quickly.

We really like cross-country skiing. We frequently recommend it to athletes with limited time who are looking for that "one good exercise" to supplement or beef up their training programs. It provides an excellent cardiovascular workout and puts all major muscle groups to work. It gets you out in the fresh air and sunshine. Additionally, it is nonimpact and easy on your joints.

After the inevitable spring thaw, you can purchase a cross-country ski machine for your den, crank up the tunes, and get in good workouts. The machines are readily available from reputable firms that will warranty them. They are inexpensive and simple to assemble, take up little space, require no electricity, and can be outfitted with all sorts of technological wonders like heart-rate monitors and mileage gauges.

It is difficult to single out muscles when describing the physiology of cross-country skiing; frankly, that's the beauty of the sport. It works virtually everything, from your buttocks and legs, which power you, to your hip flexors and thighs, which drive you forward. In the meantime, your arms are swinging, pushing, pulling, and poling from your shoulders and back. Your trunk provides stability and balance as you move along. Like an elaborate dance, everything moves rhythmically. And every move requires strength and flexibility.

Any time you will be working out in the cold, remember to warm up before you begin. A cold muscle going into a cold environment tends to contract—and fights to stay contracted, thereby irritating the attachments. Get that muscle to fire and work for you, and you'll literally feel warmer and more comfortable. Remember to drink plenty of fluids when you work out in the cold. If you associate being thirsty with being hot and sweaty, you may forget that you also need to hydrate when you are skiing. (When we speak of hydration, we are talking about water or sports drinks. Save the grog for après ski. Alcohol dehydrates you, defeating the purpose of drinking it. And, it makes you ski sloppily.) Wear eye protection, and put sunscreen on all exposed body parts. The protective atmospheric levels are diminished at the altitudes where ski runs are generally located, and you'll burn more easily than you think. A rosy glow is fine, but it should be a glow of good health, not of sun poisoning.

Cycling

Stretches:	Upper Legs, Hips, and Trunk	1–17
	Shoulders	18–27
	Neck	28–34
	Arms, Elbows, Wrists, and Hands	35–46
	Lower Legs, Ankles, and Feet	47–59

Coaches' Notes

Bicycles, tricycles, tandem bikes, road bikes, track bikes, bikes with training wheels, adult trikes, BMX bikes, mountain bikes, touring bikes, stationary bikes, recumbent bikes, unicycles . . . the list is seemingly endless, as is our fascination with the sport of cycling. It's a sport for nearly everyone. And it is a good workout.

Leg muscles are primary performers. When depressing the pedal, you use hip and knee extensors (quads) and ankle flexors (tibialis anterior). In raising the pedal, you use your hip and knee flexors (hamstrings) and ankle extensors (gastrocnemius muscles). This performance is consistent, particularly with the use of toe clips that lock the feet into position. Your arm extensors help you steer, and they support some of the weight of your trunk as you lean into the handlebars in cycling's signature aerodynamic position. But your trunk isn't just along for the ride; your back and abdominals serve as your foundation for stability—they transmit the support work of your arms to your legs. Your upper back and neck are holding your head up. (It helps to see where you are going!) Additionally, as you pump, you are getting a no-impact aerobic workout (notice, we said NO-impact).

It will come as no surprise that injury is an inherent part of cycling. The most common injuries result when a cyclist hits the pavement: road rash, cuts, bruises, and broken bones. We don't treat those injuries in our clinic. We refer them to a hospital emergency room. What we do see are overuse injuries. We can help you avoid them by advising you to train intelligently for strength and flexibility.

Cycling, as fabulous as it is, is not a perfect exercise. Pedaling around and around shortens the muscles while they work. The result? Seriously imbalanced, inflexible muscles.

The most common overuse injuries in cycling are nerve compressions of the hand (ulnar nerve) and forearm (radial distal nerve). Contracted muscles tighten up and put the nerves in a stranglehold, causing pain, numbness, fatigue, weakness, and irritation. Tight shoes, too short a distance between the seat and the pedals, too much force down on the pedal for extended periods of time, and weak muscles in the lower leg can also cause nerve compression in the foot. Flexibility training will probably cure the problem, but it may take some time before you are 100 percent. Cycling can also cause inflammation of the tendons where they attach to the hip, knee, and ankle. Overly tight quadriceps can compress the kneecap against the joint. There can be pressure on the nerves of the cervical spine at the back of the neck (from hyperextending), neck fatigue, low back pain, and pain deep in the buttocks (sciatica). Flexibility and strength will prevent all these problems.

Our advice: Sit upright from time to time and take the pressure off your back and neck. Stand up in the pedals and get the pressure off your butt. Remove your hands from the handlegrips one at a time, shake them out, and flex your fingers to get blood flowing. And remember to wear your helmet at all times. We want you to survive every little skirmish with the pavement.

Discus

Stretches:	Upper Legs, Hips, and Trunk	1–17
	Shoulders	18–27
	Neck	28–34
	Arms, Elbows, Wrists, and Hands	35–46
	Lower Legs, Ankles, and Feet	47–59

Coaches' Notes

Discus, one of our favorite sports, is one of the original five Olympic Pentathlon events and was mentioned as early as 1300 B.C. in

Homer's poetry. Few sports have such a distinguished history. Fortunately, little has changed since antiquity. When we look at today's discus thrower, we still see a solitary human being pitted against a heavy metal disk. It's so basic and simple, yet so elegant.

Discus requires incredible power. We see a lot of beginners who train with weights to become strong. That's good, but strength is only one component. You also need flexibility, to assist you in weight training more efficiently, and to help give you the body you need in order to wind up fully, toss smoothly with control, effect an adequate follow-through, and return to position on your feet. It's fascinating to watch the power explode through a discus thrower. It starts in the feet, ankles, and lower legs; travels up the legs, through the knees, up the thighs to the hips; accelerates through the trunk; and drives up through the chest and shoulder until it explodes from the arm and hand. The miracle of a discus throw is that, as you are unwinding a full body rotation, still harnessing and directing this ballistic force, suddenly you must make a decision about WHEN to release the discus. You must nail a precise moment in order to project the discus in the right direction. This "chain of command," starting with your feet and ending with your mind, requires great flexibility for a smooth and efficient transmission of all the power possible into that final release.

Most injuries in discus throwing tend to be in the wrist and hand because of the weight of the disk and athletes' mistakes in release. But the rest of the body is also susceptible to injury. It is easy to become unbalanced physically, because one side of your body works differently from the other side. We see knee injuries from torque, ankle sprains, back and neck strains, and shoulder sprains and separations. Stretching and strengthening of the entire chain of interacting muscles (both sides!) is required for you to excel at this sport and stay healthy while you enjoy it.

Fencing

Stretches:	Upper Legs, Hips, and Trunk	1–17
	Shoulders	18–27
	Neck	28–34
	Arms, Elbows, Wrists, and Hands	35–46
	Lower Legs, Ankles, and Feet	47–59

Coaches' Notes

Fencing requires lightning reflexes, superb eye–hand coordination, agility, balance, flexibility, and enormous strength to put all this together with thrust, parry, and riposte. Since the advent of electrical scoring in epee and foil competitions, fencing has evolved into a sport of speed, agility, precision, and endurance. Legs must move explosively as you go back and forth along the piste, drawing into play your hip flexors (quads), hip extensors (hamstrings and adductors), knee extensors (quads), and ankle flexors (tibialis anterior or shin muscles).

You'll use the front of your upper arm (biceps), the back of your upper arm (triceps), and your forearm, wrist, hand, and fingers in positioning the weapon arm and in stabilizing the wrist. To begin the bout (the "en garde" move), where the forearm is held upright and the weapon moves in a small circle, the muscles of the forearm rotate along a longitudinal axis (pronation and supination). Simultaneously, the muscles in the upper back (subscapularis) and the muscles in the chest (pectoralis major) perform an internal rotation. The shoulder and upper arm do an external rotation. All of these muscles must move in concert for just this one small action. It's a complicated sport.

In order of frequency, fencers injure ankles, heads (somebody's not wearing protective gear!), and hands. It makes sense that ankles are most vulnerable; they are planted, flexed, and rotated on the trail leg during high-intensity attacks and deflections. Fencers also suffer from overuse injuries such as back strains, groin pulls, ruptured Achilles tendons, and quad strains. You're out there a long time and you repeat moves endlessly.

Our words of advice: Fence ONLY with standardized equipment and ONLY with experienced opponents. Wear your protective equipment at all times, even when you're practicing. We don't want to see you in our clinic covered with little round bruises or tiny little holes. "En garde!"

Football

Stretches:	Upper Legs, Hips, and Trunk	1–17
	Shoulders	18–27
	Neck	28–34

Coaches' Notes

When we coach strength and flexibility, we are training an athlete to maximize performance and prevent injury. When we work with a football player, we are coaching to maximize performance and *minimize injury,* grudgingly acknowledging that getting hurt is almost inevitable. Football is a collision sport. It combines the athletics of track and field with the brute force of boxing or wrestling . . . or of driving an eighteen-wheeler into a brick wall at high speed! When you must get an opposing player out of your way in order to do your job, the nature of football becomes a simple question of physics: "What happens when a movable force hits an immovable object?" Aches and pains, to say the least. The good news is that the rate of injury is dropping. The evolution of helmet design, neck protection, and body padding, and new rules involving using the head as a weapon or a target have helped. But they have not eliminated injury. Football is still a bone-breaking sport—perhaps the granddaddy of them all. And maybe that's part of its appeal.

One of the great misconceptions about body mechanics is that a strong muscle is a tight muscle. Football players tend to be big men: tall, heavy, and thickly muscled. But let's run through some questions and answers:

- What happens when a tight muscle gets wrenched in tackle? It tears.

- What happens when a flexible muscle gets wrenched in that same tackle? It yields and returns to its original position.

- Can a large, strong muscle be flexible? YES! In fact, a flexible muscle can be even larger and stronger because it's easier to train and stays healthy for even more strength training.

Flexibility training should be as much a part of your football training as lifting weights and running.

Training for football should start at your feet. Your running, jumping, kicking, pivoting, stopping, and changing directions place incredible demands on your feet. And we have to admit that one environmental condition in football has increased the injury rate. Artificial turf playing fields are consistently green and beautiful and require low maintenance, but the surface is tricky. Make certain that you test and understand the "feel" of artificial turf and choose the proper shoes and cleats to deal with it. If you play on turf one weekend and grass the next, take a few minutes to "test" the field before each game. Reorient yourself to the surface and how you can move on it.

Each position places specific demands on the body, but you should be in excellent general condition before you play. You'll want to train for your job on the team, but we caution you particularly to practice tackling and being tackled before you take it onto the field . . . or opt for touch or flag football. Wear protective gear—as much of it as you can get onto your body and still move. Hydrate properly. And play with a professional athletic trainer or a medical professional who has access to a phone or two-way radio on the sideline. Not to dispute famous Green Bay Coach Vince Lombardi, but "Winning isn't the most important thing—SAFETY is."

Golf

Coaches' Notes

Most of the pain and suffering in golf is emotional—and we're not talking about the fathomless sorrow of not being able to play on a rainy day. A weekend duffer, in a fit of ecstasy over sinking a putt, may throw the putter into the air. When it returns to earth, it may home in on the top of another player's head like a heat-seeking SCUD missile. A golfer who misses a putt that was almost a "gimme" may attack a nearby oak for harboring noisy birds that shattered her concentration. The boomeranging club shaft (now an airborne lance) is a weapon that can hurt. A good round of golf offers relaxation and fellowship. Play with mature people (of any age) who have no illusions about their own ability to lick the mental and physical challenges of this complex game. Keep the competition among the players under friendly and forgiving control.

A golf swing demands a wide range of motion of multiple zones, so flexibility of all joints is essential. The areas of your body that most affect your performance are your abdominals (for stabilization), your hip and trunk, your arm and shoulder (for the golf swing), and your wrist (for grip, control, and stability). Your power starts in your feet, ankles, and lower legs, travels up your legs as you begin your torque through your knees, up your thighs, to your hips; accelerates through your trunk; and drives up through your chest and shoulder as you tightly coil to draw back and position your arms, wrists, and hands. You unwind explosively, sweeping your arms, wrists, and hands down in the controlled, graceful arc that forms your swing. Power and momentum drive your follow-through into your "reverse C." And here is a simple lesson in physics: The more flexibility you have, the farther you can bring the club away from the ball as you wind up. Increasing this range creates more club speed as you swing down and gives you more distance on your drive. And being able to sweep into your follow-through means that you have smoother control of your shot. Flexibility means more power, control, distance, and accuracy—and fewer overuse injuries.

Among professional golfers, the most common injuries are, in order of occurrence, wrist, back, hand, shoulder, and knee. Among amateur golfers, the injuries line up as lower back, elbow, wrist, shoulder, and knee. Most injuries (except those caused by stupidity) come from ineffective swing mechanics and inefficient warm-up.

A few wise words from your advisers: Have fun. If you're not relaxing, you're missing the point of the game. You're probably going to be out in the sun, so stay hydrated. If you can, leave the golf cart and walk. If you can carry or pull your own clubs, go it on your own to get a better workout. Playing golf will not give you a well-rounded workout. You'll need to augment your fitness program with other aerobic, strength, and flexibility training.

Gymnastics

Stretches:	Upper Legs, Hips, and Trunk	1–17
	Shoulders	18–27
	Neck	28–34
	Arms, Elbows, Wrists, and Hands	35–46

Coaches' Notes

It is reported that United States gymnast Mary Lou Retton prepared for her Olympic gold medal sweep by reciting a little mantra of her own before each event: "Want a ten. Get a ten." Sounds so simple, doesn't it? Want to win? Well, then win. In reality, success in gymnastics requires an early start on the training, years of top-level professional coaching, uncommon courage, discipline, and some inherent "gifts from God." Gymnasts combine dance, acrobatics, and calisthenics to create heart-stopping, gravity-defying, breathtaking moments of beauty in the sporting arena. They are among the most fit of all the athletes. Because both male and female gymnasts run the gamut from flipping to flying, it is impossible for us to make broad statements about which muscles do what and which injuries are prevalent. We *can* tell you that if you are considering gymnastics in your program, you need to be exceptionally physically fit.

There is a high rate of injury among gymnasts, brought on by the demands made on the body. The gymnast must have total control of the body at all times. This requires strength, flexibility, balance, coordination, and stamina . . . and lots of each! Upper extremity injuries are less common than those of the back, hips, legs, and feet, but even a simple upper extremity injury can delay practice and keep an athlete out of competition. Sadly, one of the most common injuries is also one of the most avoidable. An athlete who forgets to chalk or protect his or her hands tends to rip the skin in the palms. Wrists are particularly vulnerable. Pommel Horse and Vault are responsible for most wrist injuries.

Other injuries are shoulder strains, nerve impingement (where a contracted muscle cinches up and literally strangles the nerves, causing pain, fatigue, and numbness), and tendinitis (especially near a bicep) from overuse. Accidents account for some of the injuries: hitting a piece of equipment or dismounting badly, for example. Lower back, knee, ankle, and foot injuries are all too common in gymnastics and the causes are many: dismounts, tumbling, falling, leaping, and twisting.

To summarize, gymnastics are dangerous and hard on the athlete. If you are considering taking up the sport, you'll need a good gym that specializes in gymnastic training and has regulation equipment and safety equipment in place. Make certain that the coach is qualified and credentialed, and that the spotters and trainers are alert, vigilant professionals who will take good care of you. We advise you to spend a great deal of time "shopping" for the facility and training team that are right for you.

A special word of caution to female gymnasts: Allowing your body fat content to drop below 16 percent in order to achieve low body weight may cause your estrogen levels to diminish, possibly resulting in your losing estrogen's cardioprotective properties, developing amenorrhea, and running an increased risk of osteoporosis. Every woman is different, so you and your physician will want to monitor your body carefully.

Hammer Throw

Stretches:	Upper Legs, Hips, and Trunk	1–17
	Shoulders	18–27
	Arms, Elbows, Wrists, and Hands	35–46

Coaches' Notes

Hammer throw is an ancient sport that originated in Ireland about 500 B.C. The sport has continued to evolve, even in this century, as techniques improve and rules change. We've seen this event, but not up close. We prefer not to get close to people who are whirling around, and winding up to hurl a 16-pound weight into the air after they're good and dizzy.

Fortunately, technique rather than speed is emphasized to maximize centrifugal force. The hammer actually leads you in your circle. You must be strong enough to support the weight and the forces on it. And you must be flexible, quick, coordinated, balanced, and focused. The energy of your swing is transferred from powerful leg and back muscles through your hips, shoulders, and arms ahead of the hammer. If you get out of sync with the hammer, the tremendous torque generated will lead to strain in your shoulders, back, and abdominals. Counterbalancing, the necessary leaning back against the torque, puts stress on the whole body . . . and it doesn't take much at high speed for everything to go wrong.

The swing before release must be even, with the arms locked in the "X-position" and extended to prevent a "jerking" motion of the hammer. Jerking could strain the hip, back, shoulder, and neck, and (WORSE!) spoil the throw. At the same time, the swing must progressively drive upward to elevate the center of gravity. If the thrower misses this opportunity and attempts to compensate with a last-ditch wrench backward before he releases the hammer into its signature arc, he risks strains of the back of the shoulder (rhomboid), upper back (levator scapulae), and shoulder (rotator cuff).

As much as we like it, we need to remind you that hammer throw is not a complete exercise. You'll need to supplement your fitness program with flexibility and aerobic training.

Handball

Stretches:		
	Upper Legs, Hips, and Trunk	1–17
	Shoulders	18–27
	Neck	28–34
	Arms, Elbows, Wrists, and Hands	35–46
	Lower Legs, Ankles, and Feet	47–59

Coaches' Notes

Handball, high-speed and powerful, is an exhilarating yet dangerous sport. Most of the injuries are on impact with a ball, the floor, a wall, or another player.

In handball, the primary muscles used are in your arms and wrists: the elbow flexors, arm flexors, and wrist flexors. Your hip and trunk muscles contribute power, changes of direction, and balance. Your abdominal muscles and hip rotators help you change direction more quickly. Your gluteals give you the power to push off and go after the ball. Your abductors and adductors stabilize your body and give you balance. And a good, intense game will give you a great aerobic workout. Most of the injuries we see are caused by overuse of the playing arm from the shoulder to the fingertips, and are characterized by strains, sprains, fatigue, inflammation of tendons, and nerve impingement (where the muscles swell and literally strangle the nerves in the area, causing pain, limited range of motion, and numbness).

We like handball very much. It is one of those wonderful sports that requires little equipment. It can be played on an indoor court, so it's safely available at any time of the day or night, in all types of weather. Handball builds a strong, flexible athlete with quick responses, finely honed eye–hand coordination, balance, and incredible stamina. And, as long as you're not playing with one of our clients, who managed to bean his friend in the back of the head with a 90-mph ball, we think you should be fairly safe.

High Jump

Stretches:	Upper Legs, Hips, and Trunk	1–17
	Shoulders	18–27
	Lower Legs, Ankles, and Feet	47–59

Coaches' Notes

Gravity-defying high jumpers harness speed, grace, and power to do an impossible thing: soar. High jump places great demands on your body and mind, requiring speed, lightning reflexes, thunder strength, and flexibility. As you approach takeoff, you must create enough momentum to increase your acceleration forces to raise your entire body off the ground, translate your attitude from a horizontal position into a vertical position, and rotate your torso during the transition to kick up your lead leg, extend your swing leg in straddle position, and prepare your back for the "flop." This sequence requires great contractive forces of your hip flexors and back extensors, and great flexibility of your abdominals.

Injuries occur in pulling out of the centrifugal force created by the semicircle. This move is extremely hard on ankles, and we see frequent strains and sprains. Proper foot plant is critical. Another source of injuries is present when the acceleration on horizontal approach is translated into vertical lift. That required braking action places enormous stress on the fronts of the thighs (quadriceps). This can cause rupture of the patellar (kneecap) tendon (high jumpers hold the record for this!) or patella tendinitis (jumper's knee). We explain to our athletes that strong, flexible quads and hamstrings not only give them more power, but enhance their "shock-absorbing" abilities.

Another culprit in high jump injuries is fatigue, plain and simple. A tired jumper runs an increased risk of back injuries, because he or she will expend available energy in approach and takeoff, and will be unable to complete the aerial maneuvers necessary to get the body into a safe landing position.

Strength, flexibility, and adequate rest go a long way in building a successful high jumper.

Hiking

Coaches' Notes

We are sometimes asked to define the difference between hiking and walking. Easy. Hiking IS walking, but it involves covering some distance and is usually done in a rural or wilderness setting. (However, you CAN hike in the concrete canyons of a large city. More than one surly New Yorker has told us to "Take a hike, pal!") Hiking is an integral part of many other activities such as backpacking, cross-country skiing, mountaineering, and birdwatching.

Fortunately, we see fewer hiking injuries today than in the past, thanks to emerging technologies in footwear. Good running or walking shoes are fine for short hikes on easy terrain when you are carrying a little day pack. But a longer trek on rougher terrain when you are carrying a backpack requires that you wear hiking shoes or boots scientifically constructed to provide traction, support, blister control, sweat wicking, waterproofing, and comfort. A properly fitted shoe or boot will provide plenty of room for your foot and sock, and yet will be snug enough to keep your foot from sliding forward and jamming your toes during downhill hiking.

On your downhill trekking, you'll use your hip flexors, quads, calves, foot flexors and extensors, buttocks, and hip stabilizers (the adductors and abductors). Going uphill, you'll use pretty much the same roster, but the tibialis anteriors (or shin muscles) will kick in. Swinging your arms will help propel you along and stabilize you, so you'll want to stay flexible here. And speaking of stabilizing, your whole body, in dealing with uneven terrain and the sudden addition of weight, will undergo constant compensating. You may experience aches in muscles you didn't think you were using, like your abdominals, which engage to compensate for the extreme forward flexion of your back and neck from constantly watching your footing or looking up to ask, "Are we there yet?" Take it easy and stay loose.

Horseback Riding

Coaches' Notes

What's beautiful, weighs 1,200 pounds, towers over your head, wears steel-shod shoes that can crack a bone with one well-placed kick, can run you down at 40 mph, lets you sit on his or her back (sometimes), loves grain above honor, and has a brain the size of your fist? Right! HORSE! And like all things truly beautiful, a horse is also a little dangerous.

Most of the injuries we see in horseback riding take place on the human half of the duo and result from accidents. And most accidents take place among the "green horns" (cowboy talk for "beginners"). Horseback riding is twenty times more dangerous than riding on a motorcycle. Little wonder. We all *think* we know how to ride. We've seen riders a million times on the big screen. Elizabeth Taylor and Velvet. Roy Rogers and Trigger. You just climb into the saddle, masterfully seize the reins, give the horse a little nudge with your boot heels, holler "GIDDY UP!" and go. It takes only seconds to wonder how you could have been oh, so wrong.

Riding styles and equipment vary, but basically the rider is mounted in unstable equilibrium above the horse's center of gravity and mass. To counterbalance the mass and weight of the rider's body, his or her legs hang down over the horse's sides with the feet planted in the stirrups to help stabilize the rider. Leaning too far forward puts the rider at risk for rolling over the horse's shoulder if the animal stops suddenly. Leaning too far back creates the risk of a backward somersault over the horse's tail. Balance is the key. The ground is a long way down, especially for your head—which is, incidentally, positioned at the highest point on this horse–rider configuration and consequently has the farthest distance to fall. We *insist* (no discussion) that you wear a helmet at all times, no matter how short your planned ride.

Riding uses your whole body. Your hips, legs, and feet allow you to mount and dismount. They also hold you in the saddle and are used for the signals you need to direct the horse. Your back holds you erect and allows you to pivot in the saddle to change position. Your shoulders, arms, and hands balance you and allow you to operate the reins. Overuse injuries are common, especially knee and ankle strains from badly fitted stirrups and incorrect positioning of feet. Additionally, we see some quad strain from struggling to hold an upright position and from keeping the fanny from banging on the saddle by suspending it an inch or so above the leather for the duration of the entire ride. We see fatigued backs from having the buttocks pound against the saddle in hard riding. And finally, we see "saddle bootie"—sore buttocks from an unfamiliar and unfriendly seat surface.

We advise training with the best riding instructor you can find. Condition your body like an athlete. Don't assume the horse will do all your work for you. You'll ride with more control, fatigue less easily, have more fun, and look better in the saddle if you're in shape. Keep in mind that horseback riding is not a complete fitness activity, so you'll need to supplement your program with strength, flexibility, and aerobic training. Take GREAT care of your horse. And keep your equipment in as good condition as you do your horse. Enjoy your ride, Kemo Sabe.

Hurdles

Stretches:	Upper Legs, Hips, and Trunk	1–17
	Shoulders	18–27
	Neck	28–34
	Lower Legs, Ankles, and Feet	47–59

Coaches' Notes

Hurdling is running and flying. We love it, as we love all running sports, because it provides a total body workout. Lab testing of muscle activity shows that, when we run, all muscle groups get a workout, the joints of the lower extremities demonstrate increased ranges of motion, and the athlete gets an unparalleled aerobic workout. Hurdling puts icing on the cake by putting the runner in the air, adding more demand to an already demanding sport. It rarely gets any better than this.

For this sport, you must be a superior runner. Before you can fly over a hurdle, you have to get there with enough momentum to get airborne. Read carefully the sections on running, later in this section. Learn all there is to know about the mechanics of running.

Hurdling is running . . . until you encounter the hurdle in the track; then your body mechanics change. Hurdling is not jumping. It is continuing the sprint with an airborne maneuver. If you stop to convert the run into a jump, you decelerate, practically guaranteeing that you'll be on your face in just a second. To lift your lead leg (extension), you use your hip flexors and quads. Your trunk flexes the abdominals to help bring that leg up while your trail leg follows, flexed at the knee (pulled by the hamstrings) and hyperextended at the hip (pulled by the gluteals). You drive your leading leg's knee forward to spring for the push-off foot to clear the hurdle. Your hip abductors and adductors and your ankle, foot, and calf muscles give you stability. Your trunk flexes over each hurdle and then restores you to the upright position. Your neck hyperextends as you fly. Your shoulders and arms extend: the opposite arm from the lead leg is elevated and extended forward, and the other arm is hyperextended back with the trail leg. You fly and land on the ball of your foot. It is beautiful indeed.

Injuries happen when accidental impact occurs and when overuse affects the toes, feet, ankles, knee, legs, hips, and/or back. Common injuries in hurdlers are hamstring strains, groin pulls, pelvic avulsion fractures, and trailing-knee bruises (from tipping the hurdle). One of the great dangers in hurdling is that the athlete may not be able to clear the hurdle and will fall on the track entangled in the hurdle.

We've said it before, we'll say it again: Strength and flexibility go a long way in preventing injury and maximizing performance.

Ice Hockey

Stretches:	Upper Legs, Hips, and Trunk	1–17
	Shoulders	18–27
	Arms, Elbows, Wrists, and Hands	35–46
	Lower Legs, Ankles, and Feet	47–59

Coaches' Notes

One of the most common of all plays in hockey is called "Checking," but you can't fool us. We know it for what it is: "Collision." No question about it, hockey is an "in-your-face" sport, and only the fierce survive. The injury rate in hockey is nearly unparalleled, and 70 percent of the injuries are from speed-enhanced contact—sorry—"Checking." Ironically, changes in the game over the years have increased the injuries. The sport was made faster by introduction of the forward pass and the center red line. Players race each other to the end boards, straining to get to the puck first. Out-of-control collisions at breakneck speed are inevitable. Also, the evolution of the curved stick spun off a "slap shot" where the puck rockets across the ice at speeds in excess of 100 mph. And 100 mph creates airlift, so the puck is known to rise and fall, drift and curve, in dangerously unpredictable maneuvers. Everything and everyone in its path are imperiled—even the spectators, at times.

In the skating moves, the push-off position is perpendicular to the ice and creates an overall force on the lower leg of up to 140 percent of body weight. The push-off may cause hip muscle strains—specifically, of the adductors and extensors. In the wind-up phase, the swing skate touches down, placing the center of gravity directly on the side and directly in front of the ankle, and placing the ankle, knee, and hip into flexion. In the release phase, the skater contracts the buttocks, hamstrings, and calves, bringing the hip and knee toward full extension, abduction, and external rotation. In the follow-through phase, the skate completes the power push-off with full extension of the hip and knee and a final forceful extension of the ankle. In the final phase, the recovery, the hip and knee flex to about 40° and 90°, respectively, as the skater enters a crouch position.

So what can cause you problems? You have to achieve incredible speed and perform acts of acrobatic agility while your feet are virtually locked into position by the boots of your skates. There is no opportunity to flex, extend, or rotate your ankles in order to move. Your body has to find alternative maneuvers to achieve moves that a runner or jumper could do without effort. The skates put enormous stress on you.

For shooting (important if you want to score), your shoulders, arms—particularly the flexors, abductors, and adductors—and wrists will be in action as you handle your stick. You must be able to gently finesse the puck along the ice in strategic advances, and then shoot with explosive power. Both actions require great strength, control, and flexibility.

Remember to stay alert every second that you're on the ice. Getting ample rest really helps. Your own fatigue can contribute as much to an injury as will another skater's assault. Rested, you will think more clearly, make better decisions, respond faster, and keep your emotions more easily under control. Rest is the forgotten training tool. Never omit it from your regimen.

Jumping: Long Jump and Triple Jump

Stretches:	Upper Legs, Hips, and Trunk	1–17
	Shoulders	18–27
	Neck	28–34
	Lower Legs, Ankles, and Feet	47–59

Coaches' Notes

The long jump—also known as the running broad jump—is one of the five original Olympic events. Long jump is an interesting and complex sport because it demands mastery of four component parts, all of which put enormous demand on the body: approach, takeoff, flight, and landing. Triple jump, an extension of the long jump, integrates a "hop." The athlete lands on the same foot that has hit the takeoff board, then takes off on the same foot on which he or she has landed, in order to land on the opposite foot for the next jump. It sounds more complicated than it is.

In the approach for both types of jump, you have to gain enough momentum to take flight. You must be a superior sprinter, so check out our discussion of the mechanics of running on pages 154–155. Interestingly, right after takeoff, many long jumpers actually "run" in midair until they get their trailing legs to the front.

If you're a triple jumper, you are actually exaggerating the running airborne phase in your hop. Your heel strikes first in the landing, followed by a quick roll forward. Your landing foot is pulled back and put back into position, driving the opposite knee upward to gain forward momentum.

At the same time, your arms and shoulders are pumping to help you stay in balance and rhythm, and to assist your forward momentum. Your arms literally amplify the energy to propel you forward. Your back and chest are holding you in an erect, slightly forward position. Your hands are relaxed. Your head is up. And you are breathing.

In long jump, *approach* begins the moment you start toward the board. You gain momentum as you run. *Takeoff* occurs when your foot hits the ground for the last time. *Flight* is begun the moment your trailing foot breaks contact with the ground. *Landing* is defined as the instant your center of gravity passes forward of your feet or you come to rest in the pit. Both knees are partially bent to absorb the shock and prevent falling backward.

As a triple jumper, you must have perfect technique. Falling out of step will destroy your momentum. Jumping too high will destroy your distance. With each successive jump, form becomes increasingly important because you are losing momentum.

Overuse injuries are common, as they are in all runners, but jumpers have some specific problems. Falling back onto the hands—which are thrust behind to break the fall—can result in shoulder strains and sprains. Knees are at risk if the landing is ineffective. For example, if the knees are locked and straight, the jumper's center of gravity is too far behind and the landing will be too abrupt, straining the back of the knees. Uneven strides or a pit that is badly conditioned put the jumper at risk.

Jumping, whether in the long jump or triple jump, is a demanding sport, deceiving in its simplicity. To be successful, you should be a well-rounded athlete. We suggest supplemental strength training at the gym, and flexibility work. Happy landings!

Kayaking

Stretches:	Upper Legs, Hips, and Trunk	1–17
	Shoulders	18–27
	Arms, Elbows, Wrists, and Hands	35–46

Coaches' Notes

We like kayaking for a couple of reasons: first, it's great exercise for your upper body; and second, it's a great stress-buster. When you are paddling through the tough stuff, you have no time to think about anything but strategy and action. When you're paddling through the calm water, you're relaxed.

Kayaking can be learned in stages, at your own pace of progress. Start out with still water and basic moves, then advance to white water and complicated maneuvers. At any level, kayaking puts enormous strain on your body.

In paddling, your pulling arm is retroverted from a lateral position and lowered, with your elbow and wrist flexed upward. Your pushing arm is gradually extended (to match the movement of your pulling) by the back of your upper arm (tricep brachii), and raised by the muscles in the back of your shoulder (deltoids). The entire pull is supported by your trunk rotators, low in your back and hips. Your legs are extended flat out in front of you, stabilizing and supporting the action of your upper body. The ability to sit comfortably in this position requires that you have strong and flexible hip flexors.

Injuries tend to be from overuse. We see nerve impingement in the shoulders and forearms (where the muscles swell and literally strangle the nerves, causing pain and numbness). Shoulders and forearms are also vulnerable to irritated tendons, strains, and sprains. Carpal tunnel syndrome is another occupational hazard; the repetitive motion of paddling and the unyielding pressure on the hands cause fatigue, pain, numbness, and irritation. The kayaker's back is vulnerable to strains from top to bottom, with disk herniation a possibility. And the pelvis, from the kayaker's signature seating position, falls prey to tendinitis in the back of the upper legs (hamstrings), sciatic nerve compression (look for numb feet!), and various other irritations from pressure and overuse. Interestingly, we see more injuries in the early season, when kayakers are "out of practice" and when enthusiasm to hit the water leads them to skimp on warming up.

We like to warn our kayakers about the intrinsic difficulties of being cold and wet all day. Warm muscles work more efficiently and maintain flexibility longer. Cold water may, during the course of your run, compromise your warm-up and preparation efforts, so you'll want to be extra cautious. While you are paddling, scoot your bootie once in a while, to get the pressure off your lower extremities and get some blood flowing. Kayaking is not a complete exercise; you'll need to supplement your training program with some lower body work and aerobic workouts. DO NOT kayak without a helmet and life vest. We want you to rock and roll, but we want you to do it safely.

Martial Arts

Coaches' Notes

As with all combat sports, we have very mixed feelings about martial arts. We like the history—the deep roots in the philosophical Orient. We like the variety—from karate to kendo, from judo to jujitsu, from tae kwan do to Thai kick boxing. We like the discipline that forms character and infuses order in a chaotic life. We like the training that produces some of the most physically fit athletes on the planet. But what we don't like is a sport that requires a winner to beat another human being into submission. And we don't like a sport in which injuries are deliberately inflicted and cannot be avoided with proper training and conditioning. When you understand that our mission is to build and maintain superior athletes, you can easily understand the conflict we feel when we work with some martial artists.

For purposes of discussion, we deal here with basics in the training that accompany martial arts. Distance running and cycling will give you cardiovascular endurance. Wind sprints will give you fast-twitch muscle fiber conditioning and increased anaerobic capacity. Practicing on your own or with a sparring partner will increase your endurance, speed, coordination, eye–hand coordination, reflex action, striking power, and general conditioning. Strength training with light, free weights builds muscle. The benefits of a good Active-Isolated Stretching routine are increased speed and force of muscle contraction, and improved muscle memory and coordination for specific moves. Warming up is critically important; it reduces the risk of injury to a martial artist's muscles, tendons, and ligaments by elongating and bringing blood to the tissue and attachments prior to the ballistic and abrupt required movements.

Injuries include fractures of hands and feet, and nerve injuries to the hands and wrists. Most injuries occur among less experienced martial arts students who simply make mistakes. When injuries occur in experienced fighters, they are generally very serious. Mistakes are more powerfully delivered at this level.

If you are going to study martial arts, find the most qualified teacher (only a black belt, nothing less). Minimize your risks by training diligently, staying alert, sparring with partners you can trust to be responsible, and encasing yourself in as much protective gear as you can wear. With training, you'll soon be able to snatch the pebbles from our hands, Grasshopper.

Pole Vault

Coaches' Notes

Pole vaulting is one of our favorite sports because it combines the superior workout of running with upper-body-strength training. But the simple truth is: We love to see an athlete fly! Pole vaulting transforms a mere earthbound mortal into a gravity-defying aeronaut. We are endlessly surprised and thrilled by the sport.

New, lightweight Fiberglas™ poles have changed the sport of pole vaulting in two significant ways: approaches are easier and faster, and vaulters have more "spring" for catapulting. As helpful as the new pole is, it is only as good as your plant, so a proper plant is vitally important. Your plant starts with a swift, controlled run that gains you enough momentum to get you airborne, so you must be a good runner. (See our discussion on pages 154–155.) Part of your challenge as a pole vaulter is that, in normal running, your arms pump, assist your forward momentum, and counterbalance your body: your left arm moves forward with your right leg, and your right arm moves forward with your left leg. It all works very well . . . until you add an 18-foot pole that you must carry with both hands, hoisted over your head, while you rocket down the track. Your arms can't do their job and your body must compensate. We would suggest that, in training, you do some running with your hands free and your arms pumping, in order to get a good workout and prevent imbalances.

Vaulting is a complicated maneuver that fires off every muscle system in your body—starting with your legs, as you translate thundering forward momentum into powerful upward motion. Takeoff activates your chest, shoulders, and arms. When you swing and roll, your abdominals, hip and thigh flexors, and arm adductors get into the act. Extending and rotating trigger the simultaneous extension of the hip (gluteus maximus), trunk (erector spinae), and knee (quadriceps femoris). Your rotation begins when your hip reaches the level of your upper hand on the pole. Then you begin to rotate along the longitudinal axis (rotation of the trunk muscles). Simultaneously, your upper arm begins to flex and your lower arm extends. You release the pole and cross the bar when your shoulder gets higher than your upper arm. Your lower arm begins to push off from the pole, quickly followed by the upper arm. You'll be proud to know that, in these few seconds, you hold the world's record among all athletes for flexing, extending, and contracting muscles. The range of motion of a pole vaulter's lower spine has been documented with a high-speed camera to go from 40° of extension to 130° of flexion in 0.65 second. This springing action exerts tremendous stress on your back and abdominals (as well as your whole body!).

Injuries we see in pole vaulters occur from overuse and from impact (pounding the track, striking equipment, or landing badly). Shoulder injuries lead the list—ligament and muscle strains, and rotator cuff tears. Shoulder problems are followed by strains of the neck, abdominals, hips, and quadriceps—most incurred in that wrenching thrust over the bar. A word of advice about landing (besides "Do it well!"): Slap the mat hard when you land. Setting yourself up to slap snaps you into a better landing position, and the actual slapping helps to dissipate the energy of the force of your landing and decreases the chances of your hurting your back.

Race Walking

Stretches:	Upper Legs, Hips, and Trunk	1–17
	Shoulders	18–27
	Lower Legs, Ankles, and Feet	47–59

Coaches' Notes

The universal first impression of race walking is that it "looks funny," but to fitness professionals, race walking looks like a great, low-impact aerobic exercise, well suited to just about everyone. We are seeing it more and more frequently on the streets and in recreational distance road running races.

The big difference between race walking and running is that race walking has no airborne phase. When we are trying to demonstrate this difference in teaching, we take our athletes to a track and get them to walk. We trot beside them and prompt: "Walk faster. Now faster. Now faster! FASTER!" As the walkers accelerate, they reach a moment in their stride when, in order to go just that much faster, they have no choice but to pick each foot up off the ground just after a "push off." This is the second at which the walking becomes running. Try it yourself, and you'll clearly understand the difference. Race walking demands that you accelerate and gain speed, but NEVER lift that second foot off the ground. In competition, you'll be disqualified instantly if you make that forbidden transition. In recreational events like the New York City Marathon, where there are no running and walking rules, skill in race walking when you're too tired to run might allow you to rest some tired muscles for a while and still maintain forward momentum toward the finish line.

Race walking requires that you keep your body erect, with no forward lean. Your arms and upper body are used to balance, counterbalance, and amplify the movements of your hips and legs. Most athletes clench their fists, but we encourage you to try to relax your hands; it's easier on your back. Because you are essentially sprinting without the airborne phase and forward lean, your "back" leg must stay on the ground longer as you travel over it. Your ankle must dorsiflex to stay down. Your hips swing, in the gait that we consider to be the signature of race walkers.

Injuries occur because of the exaggerated amplification and stride length. For example, because the "back" leg stays on the ground, pretibial muscles in the front of the lower legs are strained, causing shin splints. Additionally, we see Achilles strains, and pain behind the knees. The extreme trunk rotation (hip swing) causes strain in the abdominals, obliques (over the ribs), lower back, and buttocks.

Race walking requires retraining your body to move in a "new" way. At first, everything will feel odd and you may experience discomfort. Flexibility is extremely important for achieving the extreme movements: walking completely upright, resisting the airborne phase of your gait, gaining and holding speed, swinging your hips, and amplifying your lower body motions with your upper body.

Race walking is interesting, but it is not a full body workout. Supplement your training with some upper and lower body work, and flexibility work. The range of movement in race walking is very limited, and you need to compensate.

A final word from your advisers: Maker certain that you have really good shoes that will provide support and cushioning. Also, remember to drink adequately. Hydration is very important. Stretch before your walk, during your walk (if you start to tighten up), and after your walk.

Racquetball

Stretches:	Upper Legs, Hips, and Trunk	1–17
	Shoulders	18–27
	Arms, Elbows, Wrists, and Hands	35–46
	Lower Legs, Ankles, and Feet	47–59

Coaches' Notes

In our clinic one afternoon, a recreational tennis player was seriously discussing leaving the sport. She hated being outside in unpredictable weather (mostly blazing heat); the sun got in her eyes and messed up some sure shots; the club dress code was getting on her nerves; she loathed "fetching" renegade balls that rocketed out of center court and came to rest in the next county; her arm and shoulder were fatigued continuously from wielding her racquet in that semilocked-elbow position; and her "Gumby" wrist kept giving way during her swing. She was fed up, but, in spite of her long list of gripes, she loved tennis. After some thought, we hit on a compromise: *racquetball,* which can be played indoors, out of the weather, and in artificial light especially designed for court illumination. No shadows. No glare. No heat. No dark. Her outfit would be of no consequence. Racquetball frequently is played on a closed, indoor court with a ceiling, four walls, and a floor, so no ball can escape without an accomplice. No chasing. The smaller, lighter, and shorter racquet would reduce the strain on her hand, wrist, arm, and shoulder. And her "Gumby" wrist would be considered a distinct advantage in the flicking and slap-action of a racquetball shot. Our client left tennis that afternoon and never looked back. Embracing racquetball, she advanced to the state championship within a year.

Racquetball is played at high speed. Just stepping onto the court raises your adrenalin and puts you on your toes. You poise and wait for the serve by crouching and balancing your weight forward, ready to spring, and alert to your opponent's slightest move. Success depends on your ability to anticipate the trajectory of a shot or bounce and to arrive in position before the ball does. We would say that there is no time to think, but, in fact, you are observing, calculating, making strategic decisions, and maneuvering in the blink of an eye. Racquetball is an amazing game that will give your whole body an amazing workout. Also, it is a guaranteed stress reducer.

We can't easily single out individual muscles when describing the physiology. If you play full-tilt, you are going to work nearly all zones, combining gymnastics, acrobatics, and racquet skills. The game requires enormous strength, flexibility, aerobic capacity, stamina, balance, eye–hand coordination, and depth perception. But, among these attributes, we find the game's dangers. Overhead strokes cause shoulder problems such as rotator cuff tendinitis and nerve impingement (where the muscle contracts and literally strangles a nerve, causing pain and numbness). Because of the racquet's light weight and the "slapping" stroke, we see elbow and wrist strains and tendinitis. Ankle and feet sprains and strains result from rapidly (and may we add, unsuccessfully) changing directions or pivoting. Most of the injuries are from accidents during the game: cuts and bruises caused by collisions between a player and the wall, an opponent, a racquet, or the ball. The most serious collision injury is one that involves eyes, so we order you to wear eye protection at all times when you play.

You will train best for racquetball if you have strength, flexibility, and aerobics programs in your workouts. Have fun!

Rock Climbing

Coaches' Notes

Even though our clinic is located in the middle of flat Manhattan, there are plenty of rock climbers right here—as there are in all parts of the world. Because of the popularity of this sport, many fitness centers are now constructing "climbing walls" in their facilities. These are multistoried, sheer-faced, simulated vertical cliffs specifically designed to offer a climber a variety of technical and strategic climbing challenges. Partly because of the climbing walls and television exposure, rock climbing is enjoying newfound popularity.

In rock climbing, size is not an issue—as long as it is matched by flexibility, strength, and stamina. Men and women do equally well, regardless of size or weight, with appropriate training. In rock climbing, *all* muscles are engaged, from the tips of your fingers to the tips of your toes, and everything in between. (This is one of the few sports that require fingers and toes to be highly conditioned.) Weight training and conscientious flexibility work are important. Additionally, you should supplement your training with aerobic workouts such as running or cycling. Rock climbing does not provide a high-quality aerobic workout, but your climb will benefit from increased endurance and ability to work at altitude if you are cardiovascularly fit.

Most injuries in rock climbing are in the hand, most commonly in the ring finger. When a climber must crimp and pull the body up on a small hold, the hand generally and that finger specifically are stressed. Injuries also occur when a climber slips and "catches" himself or herself with the hand. We are relieved to report that injuries from falling are fewer than we expected.

Equipment is crucial to the success of your climb and your personal safety. Experts advise an investment in the very best shoes and safety gear. Inspect your equipment before and after every climb. When you see something showing wear and tear, repair or replace it immediately. Train between climbs. Study with experienced teachers. Don't climb if you are not feeling 100 percent. Get plenty of rest. And be careful. We want you to live to climb another day.

Rowing/Sculling

Coaches' Notes

Our client knew instantly that he had made a *big* mistake when he signed up for sculling and checked in at the boathouse before his first class to claim his "paddle." He swears that ice actually formed on the lake in that sickening minute between his blurting out the "P" word and his daring rescue by a soon-to-be fellow oarsman who grabbed him by the sleeve and choked, "It's an OAR, you moron." More than a year later, the sculling elite from that club still call him "Pocahontas," but they *have* stopped jamming his outriggers. Forgiveness must be forthcoming.

Rowing (one oar) and sculling (two oars) put very similar demands on your body. Pulling the oars toward you against the resistance of the water, then lifting the oars and returning to position, engages the fronts of your upper arms (biceps brachi), your chest (pectoralis major), the backs of your upper arms (triceps), the backs of your shoulders (latissimus dorsi), and your upper back (teres major). While you are rowing, your trunk muscles (primarily the subscapularis) hold you erect, stabilize you, and assist you as you bend and reach. Your abdominals are used to bend forward. Your lower back (erector spinae) leans you backward. All the while, your feet are braced in the footrests, so you can flex and extend your hips, knees, and ankles as you roll your seat fore and aft, transmitting power through your whole body into your arms and the oars. Rhythm, coordination, balance, strength, flexibility, and stamina are very important.

Injuries in rowing and sculling occur most frequently in the knees. The athlete sits in a very confined position, executing very specific, repetitive movements. The knees, which power this back-and-forth action, track a very specific path. Knee irritation and overuse syndromes are common. Low back injuries follow knee problems, and are caused by pressure from the seat and exertion from the rowing. The rowing can be so strenuous, in fact, that the athlete may suffer from stress fractures of the ribs from pulling. Additionally, we see wrist and forearm irritations caused by overuse, particularly in cold weather.

Rowing is wonderful exercise, but is incomplete. Supplement your training with weight training for strength, flexibility for increased range of motion, and aerobic work for cardiovascular fitness and stamina. Allow yourself plenty of rest during preseason and during your schedule of competition. Warm up adequately before each outing. Stay hydrated and keep warm.

Rugby

Stretches:	Upper Legs, Hips, and Trunk	1–17
	Shoulders	18–27
	Neck	28–34
	Arms, Elbows, Wrists, and Hands	35–46
	Lower Legs, Ankles, and Feet	47–59

Coaches' Notes

Rugby has been described as "controlled violence." We agree that it's violent, but it looks a little out of control to us. And if any rugby player wishes to deny it, our statistics reveal that 15 percent of all injuries are from *illegal* moves. (And those are just the ones who got caught!) Rugby is a brutal competition, but who would suspect it of a sport that starts each match with both teams in the center of the field with their arms around each other?

Arms around each other is, in fact, where all the trouble begins. Right from the get-go, the scrum is a pushing, pulling, kicking bout before anyone is warmed up (not that warming up would matter much). And, if the scrum collapses, neck injuries and stompings are common. Rugby never pretended to be pretty. Even the vocabulary of this sport provides rather honest insight into the nature of the competition: "tackles," "maulings," "rucks," and "pile-ups" are fairly clear clues that rugby is not for wimps.

Most common injuries are cuts, half of which will require stitches and most of which are in the head and face. Cuts occur on impact, but we will spare you the gory details. Just picture a movable object (someone's face) meeting an immovable force (the opposing team). Following cuts are joint injuries, incurred as one player defends the ball against another player (who might be accompanied by a thundering herd). Next come neck strains, cervical spine injuries, shoulder and arm injuries, and trunk trauma.

Strength, flexibility, and cardiovascular fitness will give you some defensive tools for your own protection and some offensive tools for the success of your performance on the field. Be careful out there.

Running

Coaches' Notes

We're going to do you a major favor. In this historic literary moment, we are going to settle once and for all "The Big Argument": What is the difference between a "runner" and a "jogger"? We have researched this raging controversy from every cultural, sociological, physiological, kinesiological, psychological, and legal vantage point, and we are prepared to bring the matter to closure right now. The difference between a "runner" and a "jogger" is the fancy watch. Runner's got one. Jogger doesn't. (You're welcome.)

Let's start with the basics. Your running cadence is in three phases:

1. Foot plant (when one foot is planted on the ground and your body literally rides over the top of it);

2. Push-off (where that foot leaves the ground behind you and reaches forward to receive your weight in front of you—literally, when the back leg becomes the front leg);

3. Airborne (where both feet are off the ground, before the front foot plants again and right after the back foot pushes off).

The fact that you are totally off the ground in the airborne phase is what distinguishes running from walking.

Different parts of your lower body take responsibility for the different phases. In the foot plant phase, your ankle is the power generator, outworking your knee by 150 percent and your hip by 300 percent. (In fact, your little ankle is responsible for 60 percent of your total power in running, followed by 40 percent from the knee, and only 20 percent from the hip.) Power for your push-off phase comes primarily from your gluteus maximus.

When you run, you send 1.5 to 5 times your body weight hammering down through your legs to your feet at over 110 footstrikes per mile or 5,000 footstrikes per hour. Running places an impressive demand on your body, no question about it. But your body is remarkable in its shock-absorbing abilities. If you're like most runners, when your foot hits the track, your rear foot rolls to the inside. As the full impact of your footstrike spreads throughout your foot, your shin rotates internally, taking your foot with it, converting your foot to a shock absorber. The subtalar (the bone on top of your foot, where the ankle joins the foot) joint converts the vertical force to longitudinal force, spreading the shock through your entire foot. You adjust the torque to the surface on which you're running and then, continuing forward motion, instantaneously rotate your foot to the outside, where your foot returns to being rigid, to allow you to lift off again. It is a wonderful, miraculous process.

At the same time, your arms and shoulders are pumping to help you stay in balance and rhythm, and to assist your forward momentum. Your back and chest are holding you in an erect position. Your hands are relaxed. Your head is up. And you are breathing (very important in running).

Running provides a total body workout and a superior cardiovascular workout, but because runners are so interested in "form"—and the "form" you like is so specific—your body gets very little variety. Muscles, bones, tendons, and ligaments tend to track the same paths repeatedly. Because of this repetition, runners hold the record (70 percent) for overuse injuries among all athletes in all fields. Indeed, statistics indicate that 37 percent–56 percent of runners get hurt every year. The knees are the most common sites of injury, followed (in order) by feet, hips, upper legs and thighs, and lower back. Contributing to injury are the runners' enthusiasm and unwillingness to back off when their bodies signal that irritation is forthcoming, when running surfaces are unfamiliar and uneven, and when their shoes are worn out, are badly fitted, or are the wrong design technically and are unable to compensate for physical dysfunctions that become manifest in unbalanced footstrikes.

Strength training will help you hold your form and maintain efficiency—especially when you are tired. It will also give your muscles, bones, tendons, and ligaments some variety so that you'll be a more well-rounded athlete. Flexibility training will allow you to "flow" with a more comfortable and lengthened stride. And a lengthened stride will get you to the finish line faster, even if you change nothing else in your training program!

Some running advice: Train intelligently. The world of running is packed with excellent books and journals that provide you with inspiration, the results of the latest research, and suggested program modifications. Read them. Eat properly. Hydrate before you run. Hydrate during your run. Hydrate after you run. Stay flexible. And get an adequate amount of rest.

Running—Marathon

Coaches' Notes

The marathon originated to commemorate Phidippides, a messenger who traveled from the plains of Marathon, Greece to Athens to spread the joyful news of the victory of the Athenians against Darius the Great in 490 B.C. The problem was that it was 25 miles from Marathon to Athens. The fool was so excited that he ran all the way. He arrived, shouted, "Rejoice! We conquer!" and dropped over dead. (Anyone who has run a marathon understands why.) Today's marathon, set at 26.2 miles, is embraced by the running community as the ultimate challenge.

The basics of running are described on pages 154–155. A marathon adds an enormous fatigue factor, for which you must be prepared to compensate. This won't be your normal fatigue. This is *major* tired. The race features the famous experience of "hitting the wall," where an unconditioned body runs out of glycogen and switches fuel sources mid-stride somewhere around miles 18 to 22. (Heartbreak Hill, on the route of the Boston Marathon, has earned its name from its location at the wall.) Not only should you provide your body with sufficient glycogen to hold off the wall, but you should condition your body to run so efficiently that it will not "run out of gas" at all. And whether you "hit the wall" or just get pooped, your body mechanics will become ragged and sloppy, and a series of compensations will kick in. Typically, one of these adaptations will be the "marathon shuffle," which is characterized by a loss of length in the stride, deterioration of the gait, and flexion of the trunk (tightness in the lower back). Or, your head will fall forward, seriously fatiguing your cervical spine and upper back, which have no idea what to do with this posture over long periods of time. Or, your arms will drop and will carry your shoulders with them, constricting the chest and impeding breathing. It can turn ugly fast.

That's why your marathon training should include strength training of your upper and lower body, and flexibility to maximize range of motion. The longer your stride, the quicker you get to the finish line. In marathon running, knowing how to run is useless unless you know how to do it over 26.2 miles of pounding. Long runs in your training schedule, increased in distance incrementally over a period of time, will slowly train your body to adapt to the marathon and will give you a chance to "work the bugs out" of your run. And believe us, there will be many—running the gamut from bathroom breaks to blistering, from clothing abrasions to shoe-tying techniques.

You must learn how to properly hydrate before the race and maintain hydration during the race. When a distance runner is low on fluids, efficiency is compromised, blood volumes drop, oxygen-carrying capability is diminished, core temperature rises but there is an inability to sweat and dissipate heat, thinking becomes confused, and serious problems can set in.

Most injuries are overuse injuries—multiplied by 26.2. We see everything from strains to stress fractures. Lower body zones, starting with the pelvis, are at great risk. When you multiply the miles, injury rates rise exponentially. Seriously.

Your coaches' parting words of advice are, "Get some REST!" It is the one training component everyone ignores. Your body demands it and we are telling you to listen to that loud, clear message you're getting. Recovery helps you come back stronger for your next run. See you at the finish line!

Running—Sprinting

Stretches:	Upper Legs, Hips, and Trunk	1–17
	Shoulders	18–27
	Neck	28–34
	Arms, Elbows, Wrists, and Hands	35–46
	Lower Legs, Ankles, and Feet	47–59

Coaches' Notes

We remember one of the great international track coaches timing one of her stars, who was blazing down the backstretch of the track. The coach remarked in awe, "That little whippet was born to sprint." Our discussion of her remark after we left the meet turned into an hours-long debate: "Are sprinters born or made?" We came to the following conclusion. Indeed, many sprinters are born with inherent physical attributes that give them the talent to sprint. Muscle biopsies confirm that fast-twitch muscles give an athlete an edge in his or her ability to take a simple running gait and kick it into overdrive. Fast-twitch muscles have the short reflex times and quick reaction times that sprinters need. But, we can never discount the contribution of training. It takes *a lot of work* to be successful. (Review pages 154–155, where we discuss the mechanics of running.)

Sprinting differs from basic running in two ways: (1) it is consistently faster and (2) the basic foot position is up on the toes as opposed to heel or midsole. Sprints start from one of two positions: from running upright (such as "gunning it" near the finish line of a race, to beat another runner who pulls up beside you at the last minute) or from crouching in the starting blocks and exploding forward. Both require a push-off from the forefront of your initiating foot, a drive upward of the opposite thigh, and a quick pumping of your arms. You position your weight in front of your legs—in a "reaching" posture.

One of the real challenges in sprinting is gaining the ability to run anaerobically. We coach most runners to run aerobically—at a pace at which they can carry on a conversation—but sprinters have to perform over the threshold. Metabolites and waste products build quickly in muscles that are firing at this faster pace. Fatigue sets in, signaled by intense pain. Panting gives the runner a rapid air exchange: intake to oxygenate and exhalation to expel waste. It takes great effort. That's why you never see sprinters chatting during a race and why you see them enter into immediate recovery techniques, such as bending over and supporting their torsos with their hands on their knees, the minute they thunder over the finish line.

The most common injury among sprinters is a hamstring pull or sprain, which means their warm-up is not efficient. We also see injuries that are caused by running on the toes: calf strains, lower leg problems, and Achilles tendinitis. Banked tracks can irritate the knees; we recommend running in the opposite direction once in a while.

Strength training will help you hold your form and maintain efficiency, especially when you are tired. Additionally, it will give your muscles, bones, tendons, and ligaments some variety so that you'll be a more well-rounded athlete. Flexibility training will allow you to "flow" with a more comfortable and lengthened stride, which will get you to the finish line faster, even if you change nothing else in your training program!

We offer these words of wisdom: Prepare your muscles for action with your Active-Isolated Stretching routine before you hit the track. Drink as much as you can, train intelligently, and be really kind to your feet. Make certain that your spikes are doing their job.

Shot Put

Stretches:	Upper Legs, Hips, and Trunk	1–17
	Shoulders	18–27
	Arms, Elbows, Wrists, and Hands	35–46
	Lower Legs, Ankles, and Feet	47–59

Coaches' Notes

Putting the shot was recorded as early as 632 B.C., and, frankly, not too much has changed. We're glad. It is such a wonderfully pure sport, elegant in its simplicity. Neither high-tech equipment nor luck factor into success. Shot put pits an athlete against a single weight and truly "pushes" the human limits of strength, focus, and ability.

The space limitations of the seven-foot circle make it necessary for you to develop technique rather than speed to maximize your use of centrifugal force. You must be strong enough to support the weight and the forces on it as you circle in your low-set posture. This rotation places tremendous torque on your body. Counterbalancing, the necessary leaning back against the torque, puts additional stress on you. You must be flexible, quick, coordinated, balanced, and focused. The energy you need to put travels up through powerful feet, legs, hips, and back. When that transfer of energy hits your shoulder, it explodes through your arm. You extend and catapult the shot out and up into its trajectory arc. Simple . . . and yet terribly difficult.

Injury is caused by errors in technique. In circling and torquing, the most common injuries are muscle strain and spasms of the back. In driving the put outward, the most common injuries are strain of the buttocks and hips, and sprains of the abdominals and obliques (muscles over the ribs to the pelvis).

Workouts should include some aerobic work, because shot put provides little cardiovascular benefit. You'll also want to add some flexibility work to enhance your ability to torque, rotate from the crouch position, put, and then recover your position quickly and without injury. Weight training will help you stay balanced. Remember that shot put relies heavily on one "power leg" and one "throwing arm." The leg and arm on the other side of your body will not be as strong as your power side and will need some attention. Train under the supervision of a professional track and field coach who understands the sport and the demands it places on your body. And be smart.

Skating—Ice

Stretches:	Upper Legs, Hips, and Trunk	1–17
	Lower Legs, Ankles, and Feet	47–59
	If you speed skate:	
	Shoulders	19–27
	Arms, Elbows, Wrists, and Hands	35–46
	If you lift your partner:	
	Shoulders	19–27
	Arms, Elbows, Wrists, and Hands	35–46

Coaches' Notes

Skating is the sport that produced Bonnie Blair, whose thickly muscled body powered past her competitors like a freight train to win

Olympic gold on the speed track. Skating is also the sport that produced tiny, willowy Oksana Baiul, who danced, lighter than air, across the ice like a pixie and also went home with Olympic gold around her neck. The contrasts are sharp and the irony is intriguing. Skating is a sport that produces various results, depending on how it is practiced. Yet all skating shares some common properties.

Skating starts with balance and coordination. Because the basic building block of skating is the move forward on the ice, you begin by pushing off. One foot, at a slight angle, stabilizes. You literally press your weight against that foot while you run the other foot forward at an opposite angle. You shift your weight over the advanced foot and begin the process all over again. In stabilizing, you use the abductors in your hips, your buttocks (gluteals), thighs (quads), and calves (soleus). You flex your trunk forward, engaging your abdominals, lower back, and hip flexors and extensors to create forward thrust. For turns, you'll rely on your hip abductors and adductors. For spins, you'll use your hip and trunk rotators. For jumps, you'll stress your gluteals and abdominals. For backward movement, you'll engage neck rotators, hyperextend your hip for direction changes, and abduct and adduct your hips for propulsion. Arm and torso swinging (rhythmic side-to-side motion) is controlled by your hip rotators, abductors, and adductors, with your back and abdominals providing stabilization.

Hard workouts on the ice, placing great stress on the buttocks and legs, coupled with weight lifting with heavy plates and few reps could produce a Bonnie Blair body. Also, notice that speed skates, both boots and blades, are specifically designed to put muscles to work. In contrast, hard workouts on the ice, placing general stress on the whole body, coupled with weight lifting with lighter weights and more reps, followed by an intensive running program (to get body fat lowered) and dance training could produce an Oksana Baiul body. Notice that figure skates, with high-topped boots and short blades, are specifically designed to immobilize the ankle (restricting the work the lower leg can do) and facilitate short, quick movements.

Injuries occur differently for beginners and experts. Beginners suffer from fractures (mostly in arms, hands, and collar bones) and cuts (of the arms and hands). Experts tend to suffer from overuse injuries, most often in the lower back, resulting from improper warm-up. When an expert gets hurt, it is probably the unhappy result of a badly landed jump. The most common injuries are stress fractures of the feet and legs, bursitis, tendinitis, sprains, impingements, and dislocations. Also common are groin pulls, back strains, and fractures of the arms and wrists.

Skaters are total athletes, so your workout program should contain components of strength, flexibility, and cardiovascular conditioning.

If you're skating outdoors rather than on an enclosed rink, wear warm clothing and protective gear, such as wrist guards. Hydrate adequately. Warm up conscientiously. Skating, like all cold-weather sports, puts an extra burden on cold muscles that may warm up more slowly than you expect. Give your body a chance. Stay relaxed. Have fun. And stay out of the path of that Zamboni!

Skating—In-Line

Stretches:	Upper Legs, Hips, and Trunk	1–17
	Shoulders	18–27
	Neck	28–34
	Arms, Elbows, Wrists, and Hands	35–46
	Lower Legs, Ankles, and Feet	47–59

Coaches' Notes

In-line skating was developed by Scott and Brennan Olson of Minnesota as an off-season training tool for skiers and ice hockey players. On hills, it so closely approximates the physics of skiing that in-line skaters actually use ski poles with rubber tips. On the flats, it so closely approximates the physics of ice hockey, that you're liable to get frostbite in the heat of the summer. From the start, in-line skating was so effective and so much fun that it was embraced by recreational athletes in search of superior low-impact cardiovascular workouts. No question about it, in-line skating is the cross-trainer's dream come true. It provides low-impact, aerobic exercise; can be done almost anywhere; requires inexpensive basic equipment; and is loads of fun.

In-line skating starts with balance and coordination. Because the basic building block of in-line skating is the move forward on the pavement, you begin by pushing off. One foot at a slight angle stabilizes. You literally press your weight against that foot while you run the other foot forward at an opposite angle. You shift your weight over the advanced foot and begin the process all over again. In stabilizing, you use the abductors in your hips, your buttocks (gluteals), thighs (quads), and calves (soleus). You flex your trunk forward, engaging your abdominals, lower back, and hip flexors and extensors to create forward thrust. For turns, you'll rely on your hip abductors and adductors. For spins, you'll use your hip and trunk rotators. For jumps, you'll stress your gluteals and abdominals. For backward movement, you'll engage neck rotators, hyperextend your hip for direction changes, and abduct and adduct your hips for propulsion. Arm and torso swinging (rhythmic side-to-side motion) is controlled by your hip rotators, abductors, and adductors, with your back and abdominals providing stabilization.

Most injuries in in-line skating are the results of crashing. This sport is low-impact only on your joints; there is no pounding. But it's high impact on the ground or in the face of another skater. Padding and bracing are crucial for protecting knees, elbows, and wrists. Also, we insist that you wear a helmet. Falls and crashes are caused by uneven surfaces (the skater trips) or high speed (the skater breaks the sound barrier, but cannot find the skate's brakes). We also recommend elbow and knee pads and wrist guards.

In-line skating is a wonderful aerobic workout and lets you work your lower extremities, but your upper body is neglected. Supplement your training with general strength and flexibility, upper body work, and a little extra leg and foot work. Your skate boot restricts your foot and ankle movement, and prevents your legs from getting a complete, well-balanced workout.

Skiing

Stretches:	Upper Legs, Hips, and Trunk	1–17
	Shoulders	18–27
	Lower Legs, Ankles, and Feet	47–59

Coaches' Notes

Skiing comes in all shapes and sizes: downhill, cross-country, telemarking, jumping, acrobatic, and snowboarding. But all these shapes and sizes have one thing in common: control is gained by a single moment of weightlessness followed by a "digging in" or slipping that causes a change in direction or speed. In the achievement of this set of dynamics, the body really goes to work. Your hip extensors, knee extensors, and plantar flexors carry your lead leg forward. Your "rear" leg is carried forward by your hip flexors. Your abdominals and back support your trunk, providing stability for your leg extensors. The metatarsal arch in your foot bears your weight when you plant your foot, providing stability during any balance of weight shifts from side to side. Interestingly, the design of today's ski closely mirrors the shock-absorbing properties of the human foot: a little arch in the center which takes pounding and dissipates those forces outward. (Unlike the human foot, however, the ski cannot twist.) Your feet will be locked into rigid boots with soft, pliable linings. The boots allow limited movement of your ankles so when you decide to change the angles of your feet and skis, you must effect that change from your knees and hips, exerting force on the front and sides of your shins to translate your order-to-change down through the boots. The tibialis anterior and the triceps surae in your lower legs are also involved. You swing, lift, plant, and maneuver around your poles using your back, shoulders, arms, hands, and wrists.

Small moves make big differences, especially at high speeds. One of the signatures of a really good skier is that he or she makes it all look easy, with very controlled, yet very strong, adjustments in position. A beginner who is not quite as strong or in tune with the physics of skiing has to throw his or her whole body into a maneuver. A good example is stopping. An accomplished skier unweights the back of the skis and, with a quick pirouette of the hips, digs those skis in to "stop on a dime" and spray snow in front of the skis. A beginner must crouch down in an expansive snow plow with arms extended out to the sides and legs splayed as wide as they will go. The maneuver is slow and uncertain, and the skier is inevitably relieved when everything comes to a halt and it is possible to struggle to an upright position. As a skier improves, all movements are stronger, more subtle, and more quickly performed.

Injuries are most commonly of the knee, thumb, head, and shoulders. The majority of severe or fatal injuries result from high-speed falls and impacts. And of those, most involve inexperienced males. In fact, inexperienced skiers hold the record for all accidents: 4 to 1 over the experts.

Strength and flexibility will give you some of the skills you need to build a skier's body: powerful, controlled, quick, and balletic. At some less advanced levels, skiing is not a complete exercise, so supplement your training with some aerobic workouts. Running, cycling, or in-line skating at altitude yields superior cardiovascular benefits.

We encourage our skiers to eat properly and plenty. Skiing and coping with cold really sap your body of energy. Your body needs sufficient calories to fuel your activity and keep you warm. Additionally, we encourage you to drink water. Dehydration can creep up on you without warning. Study with qualified professionals, and master one level of skiing before you climb on the lift and challenge the next level. Mistakes in skiing can be dangerous—for you and others. Ski smart.

Soccer

Stretches:	Upper Legs, Hips, and Trunk	1–17
	Neck	28–34
	Lower Legs, Ankles, and Feet	47–59

Coaches' Notes

Soccer, the world's most popular game, is played in nearly every country on the planet. We can't decide who enjoys it more: the players or the fans. And we think both groups get good workouts during a match: the players from several hard-charging hours on the field and the fans from jumping up and down, and screaming with heart-pounding excitement.

The demands of soccer ensure that most players are in excellent physical condition with unusually refined control of their bodies. Repetitive performance of complex and ballistic movements character-izes the sport: running, jumping, rapid changing of direction, rotating, diving, heading, and throwing. Unfortunately, the very nature of these movements that sharpen up an athlete's body also puts that athlete at risk of physical injury, particularly to tendons, ligaments, and muscles that stabilize joints.

You're going to be running the equivalent of a 10K during every game, so you'll be developing the ballistic and high-speed skills of a sprinter. When you run, you send 1.5 to 5 times your body weight ham-mering down through your legs to your feet at over 110 footstrikes per mile or 5,000 footstrikes per hour. Running places an impressive de-mand on your body, but your body is remarkable in its shock-absorbing abilities. When your foot hits the field, your rear foot rolls to the inside. As the full impact of your footstrike spreads throughout your foot, your shin rotates internally, taking your foot with it, converting your foot to a shock absorber. The subtalar (the bone on top of your foot where the ankle joins the foot) joint converts the vertical force to longitudinal force, spreading the shock through your entire foot. You adjust the torque to the surface on which you're running (grass or artificial turf) and then, continuing forward motion, instantaneously rotate your foot to the outside, where your foot returns to being rigid, to allow you to lift off again. The process is wonderful, miraculous—especially in a soc-cer player, who must stop, start, and change directions hundreds of times in the course of a match.

Your arms and shoulders keep pumping to help you stay in bal-ance and rhythm, and to assist forward momentum—or to balance and counterbalance you as you quickly change direction. Your back and chest are holding you in an erect position. Your hands are relaxed. (Don't touch that ball!) Your head is up.

In soccer, most injuries occur in the lower extremities. Bruises, ligament sprains (particularly of the ankle), and muscle strains ac-count for 75 percent of all injuries. Other injuries we see are ITB syn-drome (irritation of the outside of the knee), tendinitis, and other similar overuse problems caused by high-speed changes in direction, as well as stress fractures and fractures of the tibia (shin) caused by collisions. Chronic groin pain, caused by forceful kicking, seems to be an occupational hazard. Goalies suffer from hand injuries caused by impact with the ball, the ground, or another player. An unusual injury is specific to soccer and boxing and is found in no other sports: a cyst forms in the center of the forehead, just over the bridge of the nose, caused by repeated blows to the head. Boxers get it from being struck. Soccer players get it from heading. Recent research findings from the Medical College of Virginia suggest that the cyst is not the only problem. A preliminary study of 60 players from high school, college and a professional team, who said they headed the ball more than 10 times per game, showed lower average scores on tests for attention, concentration, and overall mental functioning than other players. The conclusion may be that getting whacked in the head repeatedly causes brain damage. Be careful.

Soccer develops good athletes in all aspects but one. Because soccer is strictly a "hands-off" sport, you are missing some work on your shoulders, upper back, arms, wrists, and hands. Supplement these zones in the gym. Also, we would like to see you work overtime on developing a strong back and neck. You spend a lot of time twisting, turning, and heading. Being strong, flexible, and practiced will help you to do these with speed, skill, control, safety, and balance.

A few words of wisdom from your advisers: Stay alert to avoid injury. Like a defensive driver, you must watch out for yourself *and* everyone else. Stay hydrated with plenty of fluids before, during, and after the match. And use sunscreen. You play outside for long periods of time and you need the protection. Also, if you are offered safety equipment such as shin pads, seize the opportunity.

Squash

Stretches:	Upper Legs, Hips, and Trunk	1–17
	Arms, Elbows, Wrists, and Hands	35–46
	Lower Legs, Ankles, and Feet	47–59

Coaches' Notes

Squash has been called the fastest of all racquet sports. We are happy to note that, generally, the faster the sport, the better the workout. On the flip side of this, however, is the reality that the fast pace creates opportunities for injuries. Squash is no exception. We've heard that the sport is called "squash" because that's the sound the ball makes when it hits the wall. After working with squash players, we know for a fact that it's also the sound of a racquet bouncing off someone's head, the sound of a body careening off a concrete wall, and the sound of a ball ricocheting off a person's hindquarters.

We can't easily single out individual muscles when describing the physiology of a squash player because, if you play full-tilt, you are going to combine gymnastics, acrobatics, and racquet skills. The game requires enormous strength, flexibility, aerobic capacity, stamina, balance, eye–hand coordination, and depth perception. But, among these attributes, we find the game's dangers. Overhead strokes cause shoulder problems such as rotator cuff tendinitis and nerve impingement (where the muscle contracts and literally strangles a nerve, causing pain and numbness). Because of the racquet's light weight and the "snapping" stroke, we see elbow and wrist strains and tendinitis. Ankle and foot sprains and strains result from rapidly (and may we add, unsuccessfully) changing direction or pivoting. Bruises are common at moments of impact: player on wall or floor, racquet on player, or player on player. But, by far the most dangerous, documented injury in squash involves the eyes. Wear eye protection!

Squash is a wonderful stress-buster and workout, but it is not perfect. Only one arm, for example, is going to be worked out during the course of a game. The other will be weaker. Plan your training to make certain that both sides of your body are strong, flexible, and balanced. A squash game will give you a good aerobic workout.

Coaches' final notes: Again, wear eye protection. Warm up properly so that the sudden, ballistic movements required in squash will not damage unprepared, cold muscles. Wear shoes that will support your feet as you pivot and move from side to side. (Leave your running shoes in your workout bag; they're made for moving forward only.) Hydrate properly. And stay alert on the court.

Swimming

Stretches:	Upper Legs, Hips, and Trunk	1–17
	Shoulders	18–27
	Neck	28–34
	Arms and Wrists	35–46
	Lower Legs, Ankles, and Feet	47–59

Coaches' Notes

A few years ago, we were engaged by a swimmer who was having problems achieving performance levels that should have been well within his grasp. It was increasingly difficult to concentrate on intensifying his training that week. He turned every session into a recited litany of seemingly unrelated symptoms. He was cold. He was hot. His back hurt. His hands hurt. He had a headache. He couldn't sleep. He was sleeping too much. The list went on and on. We were unable to relate the complaints to legitimate problems and quickly got tired of listening. Then, on the third day, he said, "I had to skip lunch today. They were serving tuna fish sandwiches in the training room and I felt like a cannibal." Suddenly, we heard the cue we needed. This swimmer was overtraining. His body and his spirit were exhausted. He was in the water so much, he literally felt like a fish. So, before we canned him and threw away the opener, we pulled him off the training schedule for a few days and ordered him to rest. It did him a world of good. The point is that swimming is such a wonderful sport—low-impact and no-sweat—that it's easy to forget how demanding it is.

Swimming is the ultimate repetitive-movement sport, from kicking with legs to stroking with arms. Each movement takes place over and over and over and over . . . until something in the body becomes fatigued and starts to strain. So common is this phenomenon in swimming that we even have a syndrome known as "swimmer's shoulder"—tendinitis of the supraspinatus or biceps tendon—found in about half of all competitive swimmers. No wonder the shoulder is so susceptible to overuse injury. It is the most mobile of all the joints in the body, and yet has very little skeletal support. Strokes that are powered by the shoulder have to rely on complicated stabilizing and mobilizing relationships among the rotator cuff muscles, the shoulder capsule, tendons, bones, ligaments, and muscles of the chest and back. It doesn't take much to upset those balances. Other overuse injuries in the swimmer's body are strains, sprains, irritation, or tendinitis in the feet, ankles, knees, elbows, and back.

Although swimming is a wonderful exercise, it doesn't provide a full workout, so you should supplement your training with strength and flexibility. Also, remember that swimming isn't a load-bearing exercise—it does not put any impact on the bones. Women who rely on exercise for osteoporosis prevention need load-bearing work and should consider adding some more appropriate fitness components to their training, such as walking or running.

You may not finish a swimming workout drenched in sweat, but you *are* sweating. You're just too wet to notice. It is easy, when swimming, to forget that you need to hydrate adequately. Drink plenty of fluids. Also, look out for signs of overtraining and realize that injury is not far behind. Inability to eat tuna may be one of those signs!

Tennis

Stretches:	Upper Legs, Hips, and Trunk	1–17
	Shoulders	18–27
	Neck	28–34
	Arms, Elbows, Wrists, and Hands	35–46
	Lower Legs, Ankles, and Feet	47–59

Coaches' Notes

Tennis is one of our favorite sports. Who could resist a sport that produces such colorful characters as John McEnroe, Martina Navratilova, Andre Agassi, and Billie Jean King? Who could resist a sport resplendent with words like "love," "sweet spot," "handshake," "dink," and "advantage"? Color and charm aside, tennis is a wonderful sport—demanding, exacting, elegant, and challenging.

Part of the challenge of tennis is its choreography of instant starts, stops, leaps, pivots, and changes in direction. These high-speed ballistic maneuvers alone would tend to put a lot of stress on your body, but another part of the challenge is that, while you are ricocheting all over the court, your upper body is attacking the ball with your racket. It is a double whammy.

The most common injuries, in order of occurrence, are shoulder, back, elbow, knee, and ankle. Most injuries are the result of overuse, but in tennis overuse carries "overload"—the body can't stand up to the trauma of hard-hitting repetitive moves and develops tiny points of injury in the muscles, tendons, and ligaments. Eventually, these will manifest in tendinitis, strain, and stress fractures. In fact, one injury is so common that it is now named for the sport: "tennis elbow." Not all injuries are from overuse and overload. A little over one-third of all tennis injuries are simply traumatic: turning the ankle, tearing a knee, or fracturing a bone. We regret that injury haunts tennis, but we are heartened by the fact that most injuries can be avoided with proper warm-up, specific strength training, and flexibility work.

Avoiding injury should start with your training. Select a coach who will train you so that the dynamics of your swings and serves are perfect, and you are properly conditioned to compete at one level before you advance to the next. Select a racquet that fits your hand and provides enough weight so that you feel power, but not so much that you get fatigued easily. Go slowly at first; give your body the opportunity to adjust to the demands you will soon place on it. Your next move toward avoiding injury will be in the gym. You need a full-body workout. No aspect is more important than any other. We recommend that you organize your program to include low weights and high repetitions. You don't need bulk. You need strength. You also need a good aerobics workout. Your game might not get your heart rate up high enough or sustain it at a high rate long enough to give you maximum benefit. You need stamina and endurance, so we recommend a running, cycling, swimming, or in-line skating program as a supplement. And, flexibility is critical. You have to be able to move quickly and in control.

As a side note, please be careful when you are playing outside in heat. There is no shade on a tennis court, and the sun can be merciless.

Wear sunscreen with a high SPF, a hat, and eye protection. Also, drink plenty of fluids before, during, and after play. Carry a large bottle of water to the edge of your court and use every opportunity to sneak a sip. Also, as you are strolling to the side, use that time to swing your arms gently (get them over your head!) to give your shoulders a full range of relaxed movement without impact.

Triathlons/Biathlons

Stretches:	Upper Legs, Hips, and Trunk	1–17
	Shoulders	18–27
	Neck	28–34
	Arms, Elbows, Wrists, and Hands	35–46
	Lower Legs, Ankles, and Feet	47–59

Coaches' Notes

The triathlon is the competitive evolution of simple cross-training. And cross-training is the refuge and last resort of injured runners AND cyclists AND swimmers—any endurance athlete who can't participate in his or her own sport and seeks alternatives for training. The wonderful thing is that, when an athlete crosses over, he or she often finds another sport of equal delight and develops expertise in a second or third discipline. The advent of triathlon competitive events gave specific form to the "sport," but it is, in fact, a combination of three distinct endurance sports: swimming, cycling, and running.

At this point, we ask you to read the Coaches' Notes for swimming, cycling, and running. Triathloning is greater than the sum of its parts. There is this tricky matter of "transitioning"—performing in one sport and rapidly shifting to another. This is one of the demands of the triathlon that make it so attractive to athletes who savor a complex challenge. Not only are the logistics difficult—changing clothes and shoes and equipment while hopping through a parking lot—but the human body reacts to this madness by staging rebellion. And quelling this rebellion is the threshold issue for a successful triathlete.

Most triathlons start with a swim. Your body is horizontal; your neck is flexed; your arms are pulling; your legs are kicking from your hips with semirigid knees and relaxed feet; your back is powering the whole effort; and you are breathing hard. In fact, you are probably on the border of going anaerobic. Your body is losing heat in the cold water. Your heart is really pumping. The swim ends. You're tired. Lactic acid and other waste products from muscles firing begin to build. Too bad. You're not nearly done.

Cycling begins. You scramble out of the water on bare feet, put those wet, bare feet into shoes, perch yourself on your bike and explode out of the parking lot. No warm-up. No preparation. Now your arms, tired and pumped, are extended down as your hands clamp onto your handlegrips. Legs that were extended in the water are now required to flex and pump. And feet that were relaxed are now bearing down on the pedals. A back that was straight is now bent forward. A body that was cold in the water now heats up—a lot. The bike ride is over. Lactic acid and other waste products from muscles firing continue to build. Too bad. The worst is yet to come. You have a run to complete, and, of the three events, the physical demands of the run are the most shocking to your body.

You leap off your bike, throw yourself on the ground, change your shoes again, leap up, and start to run. No warm-up. No preparation. A back that has been bent forward is now straight up and getting pounded. Legs that have been spinning must now change pattern and bear weight—lots of it. Arms that have been frozen in a bent-elbow position on the handlegrips of your bike must now pump to help balance and propel you forward. Lactic acid and other metabolic waste make your legs feel like lead and set your arms on fire. Muscles cramp and strain. Everything hurts. You are one whipped puppy. And then, FINALLY, it's over. No wonder you love it so much. It's a GREAT sport. Exhausting, but great.

In discussing the injuries endemic to triathlons, refer to the sections on the individual sports and then add transition problems. Without warming up and preparation, going from one physical pattern to another is guaranteed to cause the body overuse, overload, and risk of traumatic injuries. You can avoid some of the problems by ensuring that you are in excellent condition before you compete. Remember that training for all three events is radically different from competing in all three in rapid succession. You probably are not doing that in training; you're cycling one day, running the next, and swimming every afternoon—or something like that. Discovering the best ways to ease your body through those transitions can add some interesting dimensions to your training and give you an edge in competition. We would like to suggest "Bricks"—training with two of the three sports back-to-back in one workout.

We caution you to train intelligently. Try to balance your skills in all three sports, so that you will not injure yourself in your "weak" sport and then injure yourself in your "strong" sport as you try to make up lost time. In competition, hydrate adequately. Because your energy expenditure is enormous in a long-distance triathlon, you might consider fueling your program—perhaps drinking an energy replacement fluid or eating a banana along the route. Remember that the purpose of triathlons is to provide a cross-training experience and that being a triathlete puts you at the top of the pack in achievement of fitness. It should be fun and you should feel great. Anything less means you're doing something wrong and need to adjust your program or your attitude. Enjoy!

Volleyball

Stretches:	Upper Legs, Hips, and Trunk	1–17
	Shoulders	18–27
	Arms, Elbows, Wrists, and Hands	35–46
	Lower Legs, Ankles, and Feet	47–59

Coaches' Notes

We have seen volleyball come full circle. It has evolved from a recreational activity to a highly competitive Olympic event, to a glitzy pro sport, and back to a popular recreational activity. Recreational volleyball delights us most.

Because the game can be staged on a variety of surfaces, players set up on uneven lawns riddled with gopher holes, beaches with deep and soft sand, or playgrounds with hard-packed dirt. And when the surfaces are unpredictable and the game is fast-moving, the result is often injury. Some studies have suggested that the harder the surface, the greater the incidence of injury. Good-quality shoes with lots of support and shock-absorbing insoles can compensate to a degree. Caution goes a long way in preventing injury.

Injuries in volleyball are most common in legs and feet. Leading the list are ankle sprains caused from leaping into the air and coming down on the outside of the foot. Sprains are followed by tendinitis, stress fractures of the shin and small bones of the foot, knee injuries, shoulder strains with nerve damage, wrist problems from badly landed dives or from setting up the ball, strained lower backs from the extreme extension and rotation required for a player to rear back and spike in midair, and hand and finger injuries from ball impact. Typical overuse injuries combine with trauma to make volleyball a little dangerous.

Knowing that most injuries are in the legs and feet will give you a clue about supplemental training. You should hit the gym and put together a program that places emphasis on your lower extremities. Additionally, you should work your back, trunk, shoulders, arms, wrists, and hands. Work with low weights and multiple reps to build strong muscles that are not bulky. You need to stay light on your feet. Also, in sports that are as ballistic and balletic as volleyball, flexibility is critical. You need to be conscientious about your stretching program. And, you will need an aerobics workout. Plan to run, cycle, swim (good for your arms and shoulders!), or skate for cardiovascular fitness and endurance.

Final words: Wear eye protection. It only takes one misplaced elbow or one rocketing ball to damage an eye. Play defensively, watching out for yourself and your fellow players. Volleyball can become a high-impact sport if you're not alert.

Walking

Coaches' Notes

A few years ago, at a small New Year's Eve gathering, a group of our friends collectively made a resolution to *get in shape*. There was much strategizing around the dinner table on this, their last night of "debauchery." By the end of the evening, everyone had vowed to hit the gym every day, run a million miles, slash calories, and eliminate all evil junk food. They made a date for Valentine's Day (six short weeks later), when they would reunite at the same dinner table and compare their glorious progress. Although we generally discourage quick-fix approaches, we endorsed the spirit of their resolution, if not their methodology. We could see some real possibilities here for all our friends but one—Glenna. She was an older woman who had never seen the inside of a gym, had never strapped on a pair of running shoes, and whose questionable eating habits were well ingrained. We noticed that she had been listening intently, but had said nothing all evening. When the group lifted their glasses to toast their New Year's Resolution pact, she had lifted hers as well. Glenna obviously wanted to be part of the group's plan to shape up. But frankly, we were concerned that our friend was in over her head, so we phoned her the next day to see if we could help. We offered to design her personal fitness program and supervise it until Valentine's Day, but Glenna politely declined our offer, "Thank you, but I'll be OK. I know what to do." We've heard that before. And we know it's the kiss of death for any fitness program. Loosely translated, it means, "I know what to do. I've always known, but never done it. And, I'm not going to do it now. Go away and leave me alone." We can take a hint. We went away and left Glenna alone. We didn't think much about it until the week before the Valentine's Day reunion. It was hard to imagine our friends all comparing their programs and successes, showing off their slimming waistlines and bulging mileage logs. And poor, soon-to-be-humiliated Glenna. The night of the reunion, everyone showed up with stories of training programs and new diets to try . . . and then there was Glenna. She hadn't been to the gym. She hadn't been on a diet. She wasn't running. But she was the *only* one with a slimming waist and a bulging mileage log. It turns out that she had been walking. Simply walking. And the results were astonishing. Most of us have been doing it since we were toddlers, are pretty good at it, and do it every day. We think of it as basic transportation, locomotion. But an intelligent few, like you and Glenna, have elevated it to exercise. And a wonderful exercise it is! Injuries in walking are few and far between. Just take it easy and increase your distance and difficulty slowly.

Walking has many virtues, but it is not the perfect exercise. You need some upper body work. Do it at the gym under trained supervision. We caution you about trying to carry handheld weights or strapping on shot-filled ankle and wrist weights. These weights change the dynamics of your stride and may cause injury by adding stress to the arm muscle attachments at the shoulder joints. It is nearly impossible to design an efficient on-the-road program that will work out all your upper body muscles, given the limitations of your upright posture and forward gait.

Invest in the best walking shoes you can afford. The faster you walk, the greater the calorie expenditure and aerobic benefit. Throw in some hills occasionally. Hydrate adequately. Warm up properly. Be careful with your headset—music is great, but you need to be able to listen for traffic and possible danger (like dogs or muggers). If you must have music, put one earphone on your ear and tuck the other one *behind* your other ear (on the side of traffic). Walk with a companion and vary your route for safety. If you walk on a path, walk the opposite way everyone else does. This will lessen the chance that someone will come up behind you. If you are going to walk on a track, walk in a counterclockwise direction in the far outside lane, leaving the inside lanes for the runners. If you hear someone coming up behind you yelling "Track!" you are being told that someone is trying to pass you. Immediately step off the track. Have a great time. If you see Glenna, tell her we said "Hello!"

Weightlifting

Coaches' Notes

One of our favorite stories about Olympic weightlifting and the "progression" approach to developing strength and musculature is

173

about Milo of Crotana, the six-time champion in the sixth century B.C. who lifted a growing calf on his shoulders every day until it was fully grown. No bull! There are ten Olympic weight categories: 52, 56, 60, 67.5, 75, 82.5, 90, 100, 110 kg, and super heavyweight (practiced without limit), and there are two competitions: snatching and jerking (neither of which is practiced with livestock). In the past ten years, it has been interesting to watch this sport reach new levels of popularity. We think it has "come into its own" because weightlifting has become a standard training tool in all disciplines of sport.

As a rule, the less experienced the lifter, the more likely an acute injury—often the result of incorrect technique, insufficient muscular preparation (too much too soon!), and inadequate warm-up. Injuries continue to decline due to high-tech, specialized power-lifting "machines" that isolate and dictate the specific tracking of a muscle and provide safety features (such as "brakes" that keep a weight from dropping onto the lifter). In addition, more educated, skilled, and experienced instructors are available.

In Olympic weightlifting, we see injuries that are both acute (like sprains) and overuse (like tendinitis). Most common are sprains, strains, and soft-tissue injuries of the lower back, shoulders, biceps, deltoids (behind the shoulders), elbows, forearms, wrists, hands, groin, thighs, and hamstrings. We know you're quickly running an inventory here and thinking that nearly every square inch of your body just might be in jeopardy. Before you panic, note something interesting. We did not mention knees, ankles, and feet. It's harder to get hurt in your lower extremities. An injury in your knee probably means you did something radically, biomechanically wrong. An injury in your ankle or foot probably means you dropped a weight on it.

We think it is highly unlikely that you would do more strength work for balance, so we're going to skip that lecture. We are, however, going to suggest that you put a flexibility workout into your training. A tight muscle takes more effort to move and can't move as fast. It will actually work against you. Also, we would like to see you develop a cardiovascular component. Weightlifting is not aerobic and you need the work.

Don't lift if you are injured or if you are not physically well. Keep your fingers as uncalloused as you are able, to avoid additional external pressure on the joints. Don't rely on your belt to give you total support. Be certain that you are muscularly developed enough—especially in your abdominal muscles—to support the weight you are lifting. Be conscientious about stretching because lifting tends to reduce your flexibility as a result of one-sided muscle hypertrophy. And always lift with a partner. (Cows don't count.)

Wind Surfing

Coaches' Notes

Wind surfing—skimming lightly along the water's silent surface with the wind captured in your sail—looks so effortless. From a distance. In truth, it is a grueling sport that requires of an athlete enormous strength, balance, flexibility, knowledge of wind and water, and hair-trigger reflexes. Otherwise, the surfer becomes a swimmer and that's another sport altogether.

As the wind shifts, wind surfing involves quick changes, which require midsection stability and upper-body strength and flexibility. In lifting and pulling the sail toward you against the resistance of the wind and the water, you engage the fronts of your upper arms (biceps brachi), chest (pectoralis major), backs of your upper arms (triceps), backs of your shoulders (latissimus dorsi), and upper back (rhomboids, teres major). While you are maneuvering, your trunk muscles (primarily the subscapularis) hold you erect, stabilize you, and assist you as you bend and reach. Your abdominals are used to bend forward. Your lower back (erector spinae) leans you backward. All the while, your feet are braced on the board with your toes gripping the surface, so you can flex and extend your hips, knees, and ankles as you match and counterbalance the pitch and roll of your board, transmitting power through your whole body into your arms and the sail. Everything is in motion, so constant changes in these muscle groupings are required.

Fortunately, injuries in wind surfing are few. And most are related to straining to pull the sail out of the water and get the board into position, and overuse of shoulders, arms, and back from controlling the sail once the board is in motion. Traumatic injuries occur when the surfer is wrenched by a sudden shift in the wind or falls. Sunburn is listed as the primary hazard of wind surfing. Because the athlete is wet and moving in the wind, the body surface is naturally cooled. It is easy to forget the searing sun just overhead. The long-term risk of skin cancer is very real. We suggest that you liberally apply waterproof sunscreens with high SPFs before beginning the day, and reapply when opportunity allows. We also suggest that you wear shatterproof sunglasses that filter out damaging sun.

There is some difficulty in being wet all the time. Hands and feet that are soaked in salt water are soon devoid of their natural oils.

Waterlogged skin soon becomes prunelike. The combination of the two—no oils and wrinkled surfaces—makes skin easy to damage. Hands that grip the rail and feet that grip the board may develop painful cracks and pressure points. Liberal application of lotion or oil after you have dried off at the end of the day, or wearing gloves and booties may help prevent small, uncomfortable injuries.

As in all water sports, it is important that you be a strong swimmer. Wind is a fickle partner and, if you're stranded in still water far from shore, we want you to be able to get back on terra firma. Take a few minutes before you start the day and swim a few laps. It will help you warm up and hone your swimming skills. A few more laps at the end of the day will help you "work the kinks out." Also, wind surfing is a good exercise, but not perfect. We suggest that you organize a workout program for yourself that includes strength, flexibility and cardiovascular training. You'll be more effective on the board and will feel better.

Drink as much as you are able. It is easy to forget that you need water when you are in water. Avoid alcohol; it dehydrates you and makes you stupid. We want you to be safe. Wear your flotation vest at all times. Tell someone when you are going out on the water and when you will return—sort of like filing a flight plan. If you have an emergency, it will be comforting to know that someone will come and look for you after a specified hour. Wear a waterproof watch, and have a great time!

Wrestling

Stretches:	Upper Legs, Hips, and Trunk	1–17
	Shoulders	18–27
	Neck	28–34
	Arms, Elbows, Wrists, and Hands	35–46
	Lower Legs, Ankles, and Feet	47–59

Coaches' Notes

Wrestling holds a few records. It is one of the world's oldest competitive sports, and it is practiced in all countries. (We're so proud!) And a U.S. National Collegiate Athletic Association five-year study rated it as having the highest injury rate of all sports surveyed. (We're not so proud.) In a high school study, injury rates among wrestlers were second only to those of football players. (We're not proud at all.)

Most common injuries occur (in order) in the knee, head, neck and face, shoulder, trunk and back, and ankle. Attacking wrestlers have more neck injuries. Defending wrestlers have more knee injuries. The high injury rate is simple to explain. Wrestling is a contact sport in which the opponents are locked together continuously. (Even in boxing, the combatants separate as they circle one another.) And, wrestling is an impact sport with takedowns (the attacking wrestler puts the defender on the mat). Even a move that is strictly by-the-book can become dangerous when it is executed explosively or is countered or partially countered by an opponent. And here's some more bad news. Wrestlers who get hurt once are twice as prone to injury after they've healed. And more bad news: Overly zealous wrestlers are notorious for not following instructions in healing and rehabilitation.

The self-governing rules of wrestling help reduce injury rates. Wrestlers battle wrestlers of similar weight, so one may not overpower the other with size. There are specific regulations regarding the placement of mats, scoreboards, and tables so the wrestling area is safe. Trained medical personnel are on duty at all events. Illegal techniques and dangerous moves are outlawed. Many organizations require protective gear such as mouthpieces, helmets, and knee pads. It is not uncommon for an organization to have regulations regarding daily laundering of clothing, frequent showering for wrestlers, and disinfecting mats to minimize skin problems such as staph, strep, and herpetic infections. In fact, a wrestler may be disqualified from a match if he is found to have dermatological problems. Wrestlers' contact is skin-to-skin, and communicable infections are easily spread and potentially very dangerous.

Intelligent training pays off for a wrestler. Flexibility is critical. A muscle that has a limited range of motion is prone to straining and spraining. We recommend a comprehensive program with specific emphasis on the shoulders, groin, hamstrings, and lower back. Strength is important for the power it takes to handle your opponent and win. Cardiovascular work will give you the stamina you need to work at maximum performance throughout the match. You need to put together a training regimen that will combine strength work in the gym and a good aerobics program.

A little more advice: There is a lot of pressure on you to "make weight" so you can wrestle as small an opponent as possible. Wrestlers sometimes do psycho things to get their weights down. Before competitions, we've seen starvation diets and guys who sat for hours in saunas without drinking water, to "sweat it out." You might be able to drop a few pounds fast, but your muscles and all the systems that drive your body need fuel and hydration in order to work properly. If you deprive yourself of necessary food and water, your body can't do its jobs. You'll pay for it with diminished strength and endurance—guaranteed. If you think you can quickly drop weight, weigh in, and then eat and drink like crazy to make up the differences before your match, think again. It takes up to 48 hours to replenish glycogen stores in your muscles, and 24 to 36 hours to recover from dehydration. You just don't have the time. A smarter approach is to be well-trained so you can wrestle someone your own weight.

Occupational Activities

Driving

Coaches' Notes

We once had a client hobble into our clinic, so locked up that he literally was unable to move his head from side to side. He was sheet-white and obviously in great pain. We leaped to his assistance.

"What happened?!?" we demanded to know.

"Car," he whispered.

"What did it do? Run over you? Hit you? Back you into a brick wall?"

"No. Drove it from L.A. to New York. Record time. Hurt me."

It sure did. We were standing in front of a classic overuse injury— of the *entire body*. He was bent over like a troll.

Driving is a great pleasure for most of us. The hours zip by as fast as the scenery. But before we realize it, we have been sitting, possibly tense, belted into one position for hours, with our arms extended in front of us and our eyes glued to the road ahead. We even have mirrors so that we occasionally can scope out our surroundings without having to move. All the controls for all the equipment are within inches of our hands or feet so we don't have to reach. All the fast-food restaurants along major highways have drive-through windows, so we don't have to get up and walk, even for food. And today's cars get super gas mileage, so refueling is infrequent. If it were not for the fact that "nature calls" us from time to time, we might never get out of the vehicle. Everything seems to be so efficient. And it is, except for sustaining life as we know it.

The sitting position puts more stress on your lower spine than standing. And, no matter how ergonomically designed and seemingly comfortable your seat is, your back, hips, legs, and buttocks are going to fatigue and tighten up if you don't give them a break. Whether you are driving a passenger car, an eighteen-wheel rig, or a high-performance race car, remember to MOVE occasionally.

180

Sitting All Day

Coaches' Notes

We once had a client call us and shout that he needed immediate help because his job was killing his body and he didn't think he could last much longer. Concerned, we inquired, "What do you do?" We were thinking, "Matador? Overly enthusiastic blood donor? Gladiator?" When he told us that he was a writer who sat at his desk all day, we were a little confused. Frankly, that sounded pretty cushy to us. How bad could it be? Within the hour, we knew. Bad. Really bad. The client was locked up from the top of his head to the tips of his toes.

Sitting at a desk all day can take a terrible toll on an unprepared body, putting more stress on your lower spine than standing. And, no matter how ergonomically designed and seemingly comfortable your chair is, your back, hips, legs, and buttocks are going to fatigue and tighten up if you don't give them a break.

The other problem with sitting is that all your work is contained within a small, specific space—usually right in front and just below your face, on a desk. Your arms and hands are usually up on the desk, and your neck is flexed downward toward your work. This is a bad situation made even worse by the fact that you lock into this position and move very little and very infrequently. Your shoulders and the area between your shoulder blades fatigue and strain as you maintain and sustain this posture.

There is only one answer. MOVE! Use every excuse you can find to stand up and move around. File things. Drop things and then get up to retrieve them. Walk down the hall to answer a question rather than use the phone. If it is inappropriate for you to stand, wiggle and flex while seated. Shrug your shoulders. Hold your arms over your head. Extend your legs out, rotate your ankles and feet, crunch your toes up and then relax them . . . do *anything* that gets blood flowing. Use your breaks and lunchtime to walk and relax your shoulders and back.

Working at your desk all day means that you are not getting enough exercise. Put together an after-work fitness program that combines strength, flexibility, and aerobic work.

Standing All Day

Coaches' Notes

If you think that standing all day is easy, just ask the Royal Guards at Buckingham Palace. More than once, we've seen a film clip of one of them as he pitched forward in a dead faint (but still at full attention).

Although we assume that you don't have to stand at attention all day, we also assume that you are upright and on your feet. When you put weight on a foot, you literally convert it to a shock absorber. The subtalar (the bone on top of your foot where the ankle joins the foot) joint converts the vertical force of your weight to longitudinal force, spreading the shock through your entire foot. Your arch is like a spring, flattening out when it is pressured and then becoming rigid again when your weight is shifted off your foot. It's really quite remarkable. But it can tire a foot when the day is long.

Another problem with being on your feet all day is that your circulation may be "sluggish." Gravity and inactivity take their toll. Metabolic wastes from firing muscles in lower extremities may not be flushed sufficiently. Fluids may accumulate in muscles and around joints, and you may find yourself with swollen knees, ankles, and feet. When tissues swell, they compress nerves and you may experience some irritation or aching. The fainting Palace Guard reminds us that your blood supply may tend to favor your lower extremities when you stand for long periods of time. Gravity, remember? When blood does not make its way back to your brain in sufficient amounts, you black out. Getting your heart pumping and your blood circulating properly usually is a simple matter of moving. However, if you feel that you are past the point of no return ("Timber!"), sit down and put your head between your knees, or lie down and elevate your feet. This will put gravity on your head's side and allow easier blood flow to your brain, restoring your sense of well-being. Don't be embarrassed. It has happened to the best of us.

Your hips and back may become fatigued from holding you in the upright position and stabilizing your carriage. You may experience some discomfort and straining.

We can't say enough about the importance of good footwear. Whether you are wearing shoes or boots, make certain that they fit properly and provide support and cushioning appropriate to your job and the surface on which you must function.

Standing all day may not provide you with a balanced fitness program, so put together a program that includes strength, flexibility, and aerobic work. Resist the temptation to skip working out your feet and legs. Standing provides a limited range of motion and is just ONE of the many functions for which feet and legs are valuable. Being fit will help you withstand the rigors of standing.

Lifting and Hauling All Day

Stretches:	Upper Legs, Hips, and Trunk	1–17
	Shoulders	18–27
	Neck	28–34
	Arms, Elbows, Wrists, and Hands	35–46
	Lower Legs, Ankles, and Feet	47–59

Coaches' Notes

Recently, we had the opportunity to work with a circus "strong man"—a huge, heavily muscled fellow who made his living by lifting bar bells nightly in front of an admiring audience. He came to us when he woke up one morning to find that he could no longer lift. We evaluated him and discovered that this giant was actually quite weak. How could a professional "strong man" be weak? Easy.

He lifted all his weights in front of his body. His backside, imbalanced and weaker than his frontside, struggled to participate in the lifting. His back, buttocks, and hamstrings stayed continuously contracted, impinging nerves and shorting out, getting weaker and even more imbalanced with every lift, until things started shutting down. When his back could no longer assist, muscles in the front had to work harder. But they weren't strong enough. And he started having difficulties with muscles in his arms and shoulders. From that point forward, his lifting days were numbered until he put in some time at the gym.

It is very difficult to look at a person who lifts and hauls and conclude that he or she is not fit, but we know that it is frequently true. When we define "fitness," we say it is comprised of health, strength, cardiovascular fitness (endurance), and flexibility. The great irony of being a person who lifts and hauls is that you may have only ONE of the components: strength. You look great, but you may be in lousy shape. To excel in your profession and stay healthy, your goal should be to put all the fitness pieces in place.

In lifting and hauling, we see injuries that are both acute (like sprains) and overuse (like tendinitis). Most common are sprains, strains, and soft-tissue injuries of the lower back, shoulders, biceps, deltoids (behind the shoulders), elbows, forearms, wrists, hands, groin, thighs, and hamstrings. Are you quickly running an inventory here and thinking that nearly every square inch of your body just might be in jeopardy? Before you panic, note something interesting. We did not mention knees, ankles, and feet. It's harder to get hurt in your lower extremities. An injury in your knee probably means you did something radically, biomechanically wrong. An injury in your ankle or foot probably means you dropped a crate on it.

Don't lift and haul if you are injured or if you are not physically well. Don't rely on a back belt to give you support. Wear gloves to protect your hands. Be certain that you are muscularly developed enough—especially in your abdominal muscles—to support the weight you are lifting. Be conscientious about stretching. Lifting tends to reduce your flexibility as a result of one-sided muscle hypertrophy. (That is, each muscle might get a good workout as you lift, but might not get a workout as you put the weight down. Consequently, the muscle develops only half its functional strength. In other words, the muscle might be great at flexing and lousy at extending.)

No matter how much you lift and haul during the day, you need strength work for balance. (Remember that lifting and hauling are accomplished from the front and there's another whole side of you!) Also, place an Active-Isolated Stretching workout into your training. A tight muscle takes more effort to move and can't move as fast. It will actually work against you. Also, we would like to see you develop a cardiovascular component. Lifting and hauling are not aerobic, and you need the work.

Pushing and Pulling All Day

Stretches:	Upper Legs, Hips, and Trunk	1–17
	Shoulders	18–27
	Neck	28–34
	Arms, Elbows, Wrists, and Hands	35–46
	Lower Legs, Ankles, and Feet	47–59

Coaches' Notes

One of our favorite clients is a piano mover who insists on "doing it himself." When he first came to us, his body was pretty beaten up. We asked him if a piano had rolled over him. "No," he grinned. "Getting banged up is part of the job. Got to get me old shoulder in there, you know." We still laugh about "me old shoulder." What was he doing that was so damaging? Throwing his whole body against a rolling piano like a battering ram—a practice common when muscles are too weak to do their jobs.

We like to send a professional out to do a really physical job with a few basics in place. First, get in great shape and stay there. Second, get yourself a firm grasp of physics: how things move and how you can move with them. Third, pay attention to the veterans who have tricks up their sleeves for getting the job done with minimum wear and tear on the body (without having to "get me old shoulder in there"). We like to advise our clients to explore protective clothing, equipment, or tools that could assist in a highly physically demanding situation.

Pushing and pulling engage the fronts of your upper arms (biceps brachi), chest (pectoralis major), backs of your upper arms (triceps), backs of your shoulders (latissimus dorsi), and upper back (rhomboids, teres major). While you are positioning your body, your trunk muscles (primarily the subscapularis) hold you erect, stabilize you, and assist you as you bend and reach. Your abdominals are used to bend forward. Your lower back (erector spinae) leans you backward. All the while, your feet are braced so you can flex and extend your hips, knees, and ankles as you balance, transmitting power through your whole body into your arms and hands. It seems to be a full body workout.

Unfortunately, fitness is not as easy as working eight hours at a physically demanding job. No matter how much you push and pull during the day, you need strength work for balance. Also, an Active-Isolated Stretching workout should be part of your training. A tight muscle takes more effort to move and can't move as fast. It will actually work against you. Develop a cardiovascular component. Pushing and pulling are not aerobic and you need the work.

Keyboarding All Day

Stretches:	Upper Legs, Hips, and Trunk	1–17
	Shoulders	18–27
	Neck	28–34
	Arms, Elbows, Wrists, and Hands	35–46
	Lower Legs, Ankles, and Feet	47–59

Coaches' Notes

We have a riddle for you. What debilitating injury, in the past few years, has nearly dominated workplace physical therapy practices? The cast and brace industry is booming, enjoying astronomical gains in sales because of it. This injury is so common that everyone knows the medical terminology for it. This injury is so dreaded and feared that equipment to protect against it is sold in every office supply store on the planet. What is it?

The reference to an "office supply store" should have given it away. If you guessed "carpal tunnel syndrome," you guessed right. With the computer keyboard firmly implanted in our technologically advancing society, carpal tunnel syndrome has become epidemic. But, you argue, keyboards have been around forever. Why are we seeing carpal tunnel syndrome now? Easy to answer. The old-style typewriter keys were harder to strike, so the hand got a better workout. And the carriage return made it necessary for the typist to reach up and whack it at the end of every line. The computer keyboard has a soft touch, so the hand must work more subtly. And there is no carriage return; consequently, there is no reason to change position. Additionally, computer work can be rivetingly interesting. It is easy to sit, locked into one position, and stare at the screen for hours.

At the risk of becoming the least popular people in the world, we are going to say something that will infuriate keyboard users and carpal tunnel syndrome sufferers. Carpal tunnel syndrome is a classic overuse injury. It is predictable and preventable. It happens when a keyboarder does not pay attention to the clear signals the body sends, the first of which is fatigue. Prevention is a matter of keeping the hands and wrists strong and flexible. A preventive measure as basic and simple as breaking the routine that causes the strain—taking a short break every hour to improve circulation, change position, and restore joint range of motion—goes a long way in making sure you don't get hurt. Copy the hand and wrist routines from Active-Isolated Stretching, and tape the pages to your monitor as a reminder that you need to train like an athlete if you're going to stress your body to this extent.

In case you thought carpal tunnel syndrome was the only peril of keyboarding, think again. Sitting at a keyboard all day can take a terrible toll on an unprepared body, putting more stress on your lower spine than standing. And, no matter how ergonomically designed and seemingly comfortable your chair is, your back, hips, legs, and buttocks are going to fatigue and tighten up if you don't give them a break. Your neck, shoulders, and the area between your shoulder blades fatigue and strain as you maintain and sustain an upright posture. There is only one answer. MOVE! Use every excuse you can find to stand up and move around.

Working at a keyboard all days means that you are not getting enough exercise, so put together an after-work fitness program that combines strength, flexibility, and aerobic work.

Part III
Stretching for Life

Active-Isolated Stretching for Expectant Moms

We got a phone call from a well-known female tennis player who breathlessly informed us that she needed to "change gears" immediately and required our assistance to revamp her training program. We agreed to meet with her and her coach—who happened also to be her husband—the next day. It sounded like "business as usual" for the Whartons, but hers was a phone call that would launch us on an unusual odyssey of adventure and discovery.

From the moment when she and her coach settled into their chairs, it was obvious that we four were dealing with an extraordinary situation.

US: So what's this all about? New play tactics?
THEM: (*Giggling*) No, it's way too late for that!
US: New sport altogether?
THEM: (*Choking with laughter*) Yeah. Sort of marathoning.
US: (*Turning to the coach*) Forgive us for asking, but are you a tennis coach or a marathon coach?
THEM: (*Exploding into hysteria*) Try "LAMAZE"! We're having a baby!

Like all people who are this much in love, they were both adorable and annoying. But once we were in on the inside joke, we understood instantly why trainers had been brought in to assist. We also had to admit that, to our knowledge, we had never worked with a pregnant athlete. Always up for a new experience, however, we accepted their challenge. At the end of our months together, we had a library full of research material—and they had a beautiful 7-pound, 8-ounce baby girl (who totally blew our vote for the name "James Phillip").

EXERCISE DURING PREGNANCY

According to the American College of Obstetricians and Gynecologists, exercise during pregnancy, within safe limits, is good for most expectant mothers—for stronger posture, an enhanced sense of well-being, easing of some of the discomforts of pregnancy such as backaches and fatigue, and preparing mom for the rigors of labor and delivery. Recent research on the responses of moms and unborn children to exercise has significantly increased our understanding of the benefits and risks. And the news is good. Reassuring results strongly suggest that exercise poses minimal risks for you and your baby. You will be less efficient in your workout, of course, because your cardiovascular system is working for two. Your oxygen requirements will be higher, and you'll find yourself huffing and puffing sooner. You're heavier and more cumbersome than you're accustomed to being. Your center of gravity is more forward. Your joints are lax. And you may be struggling to overcome generalized fatigue. Granted, the training responses and results you recognize and expect may be compromised during pregnancy, but exercise, even under these conditions, is good for you. As for your baby, he or she may experience transient effects from your workout, but there appears to be no direct clinical evidence that exercise will harm your little one—provided that your workout is safe, protects your baby from extreme heat, and does not deplete your calories or fluids to the point where your baby is being deprived. As soon as your physician gives you permission to exercise and approves your program, get back to it.

When you're pregnant, you have to deal with and adjust to rapid and radical changes in your body at the same time you should be training like an athlete for a major endurance event: labor, delivery, recovery, and eighteen years of child rearing. The combination of training challenges is formidable and joyful.

As Your Body Changes

From an athlete's point of view, the first issue is a rapid weight gain. No extra weight is easy to carry, but the weight of a baby is particularly difficult. Not only is the weight gain rapid, but it is carried in front of you. And your little bundle of joy displaces internal organs and puts pressure on places you didn't even know existed.

This weight in front of you places enormous stress on your back, particularly if your abdominal muscles are weak. In early pregnancy, your pelvis supports the baby's weight. But when the wee one gets big enough to bulge out in front of your hips, the pull forward is significant if you're not strong enough to use your abdominal muscles to snug the baby back into that natural cradle of your pelvis. Compensation for an inability to support the weight causes that signature swayback that we commonly associate with pregnant women. At this point, some moms experience pressure and aching in their lower backs, hips, and buttocks when their babies shift position and compress nerves in the moms' backs.

A Time of Flexibility

The time for getting strong is before you get pregnant, but there is much you can do to help your body adjust to this weight gain as you go along. Active-Isolated Stretching just might be the perfect workout for easing a back that is struggling to compensate for rapid weight gain and gravity shift. During pregnancy, you're more flexible than usual anyway, so you might as well take advantage of it.

As your pregnancy progresses, your body produces a hormone called "relaxin," which has several functions researchers have been able to identify. One is to help you hold your baby in your uterus. Under other circumstances, if a muscle such as a uterine muscle were stretched and stressed, it would cramp. But cramping in the uterus would make it an impossible environment for a baby. Relaxin eases the uterus (except for an occasional friendly Braxton-Hicks contraction) until it is time to deliver your baby, and then regulates fine control of uterine contractions during and after delivery. Another function of relaxin is to soften the connective tissues in the cervix and the pelvic ligaments. Literally, you temporarily get loose in the joints during your pregnancy. When the joints in your pelvis begin to relax, you may identify this as the moment you develop "the waddle." We see it as the moment you seize the opportunity to recruit Mother Nature as your training partner in Active-Isolated Stretching. Move now, and you can make some clear gains in flexibility. Here is how you begin:

- *Clear your program with your physician.* Show him or her your workout, and get a blessing before you begin.

- *Dress comfortably.* Wear cool, lightweight, loose clothing that will allow you to move without cramping your style. Your shoes, as always, should be flat, fit well, and be securely fastened. We want NO slipping. Remember that your center of gravity is adjusted. Even our most accomplished athletes report that, during pregnancy, they feel heavy, clumsy, and unbalanced. It takes only a momentary lapse in judgment to result in a slip or fall.

- *Choose a workout surface that is comfortable.* We suggest a carpeted floor or a hardwood or tiled floor over which you have thrown a mat or a folded beach towel. Again, we want you safe and cozy.

- *Regulate the temperature.* Make certain that you set the thermostat to keep you warm enough to be relaxed and yet cool enough to protect your baby from difficulties that may arise from being overheated. Under NO circumstances should you work out in the blazing heat of the noonday sun, in a sauna, or in a steamroom.

- *Stay alert for signals that tell you enough is enough.* Pay attention to warning signs such as pain, a persistent cramp or stitch, dizziness, rapid pulse, irregular heartbeat, breathlessness, numbness, sudden fatigue, headache, discharge of amniotic fluid or blood, a decrease in your baby's movement, or any potential symptom that your physician may suggest as being dangerous. If you experience anything unusual, stop working out immediately and phone your physician.

- *Expect to continuously adjust your program.* As your body changes, you may have to adjust or eliminate some stretches that will first become uncomfortable and then physically impossible. For example, when your baby gets a little heavier, lying on your back will cause the little guy to rest on a nerve in your back and cause you discomfort.

- *Take 30 minutes a day for yourself.* Try to find 30 consecutive minutes every day to work out. Think of it not as an indulgence, but as your training—a necessary investment in a successful pregnancy, strong delivery, and rapid recovery.

YOUR ACTIVE-ISOLATED STRETCHING ROUTINE

As your pregnancy progresses, your ability to move and maneuver will become more difficult. Daily, your abdominal muscles continue to elongate over your expanding belly, making it difficult for you to contract them. Eventually, when the expansion becomes extreme, these muscles separate from top to bottom along the center line of your navel. Activities that were easy for you a few months ago—like using your abdominal muscles to pull you from a reclining position to a sitting one—are nearly impossible. Later in your pregnancy, your baby literally gets in the way of some activities. For example, during your first month of pregnancy, you easily can lift your knee straight up toward your chin and snug your quad up against your body. Later, your baby's position and expanding size will make this impossible.

As you and your baby advance through pregnancy, you may have to modify or eliminate specific Active-Isolated Stretches. Everyone is different, so the decisions are individual. Continue to include a stretch ONLY if you are comfortable. Try to complete a full routine every day, but if you run out of time (or energy), we have designed a special shortened program just for you.

Stretches Guaranteed to Ease Your Back

Theses stretches are taken from the Active-Isolated Stretching program, but they have been modified so that you can work out in a comfortable position. If you are interested in learning more about each stretch, such as the names of the stretching and contracting muscles or how a stretch might be assisted by another person, refer to the full description of the stretch in Part I of this book.

Double Leg Pelvic Tilt

Lie on your back on a comfortable surface, such as your bed or a carpeted floor. Begin with both knees bent and your feet flat on the surface on which you are lying. Place your hands behind your knees/thighs to prevent pressure on the knees and provide a little assistance toward the end of the free movement. Using your abdominals and quadriceps, lift your legs toward your chest, aiming your knees toward the outside of your shoulders until you can go no farther. Gently assist at the end of the stretch with your hands, but do not pull. Hold each stretch 1 to 2 seconds, and then return to the resting position. Do 8 to 10 repetitions. You'll feel this stretch in your lower back, around your belt line.

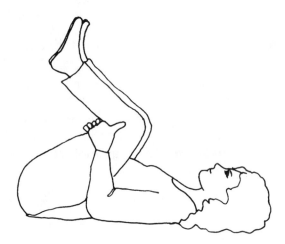

Medial Hip Rotators

Sit in a chair with your spine against the back of the chair. Place a small, rolled towel between your beltline and the chair back. Take hold of the foot of the leg to be exercised and place it on top of the thigh of the opposite leg, resting your ankle just above your knee. You may want to place a folded towel on the top of your thigh, under the ankle of your exercising leg. Contract the working muscles in your hip and outer thigh, and lower your knee toward the floor. Using your nonexercising leg as a fulcrum, gently press your knee down with the hand on the same side, and stabilize and assist the stretch with your opposite hand by grasping your foot. Work one side at a time. Hold each stretch 1 to 2 seconds, and then return to the resting position. Do 8 to 10 repetitions. You'll feel this stretch in your outer hip and inner thigh.

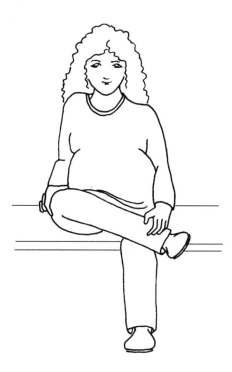

Trunk Extensors

Sit on the edge of a chair with your back straight and your feet flat on the floor, shoulder width apart. Tuck your chin down, contract your abdominal muscles, and pull your body forward until your head is well below your knees. Grasp the sides of your lower legs with your hands to gently assist at the end of the stretch. Hold each stretch 1 to 2 seconds, and then return to the resting position. Do 8 to 10 repetitions. You'll feel this stretch in your lower back.

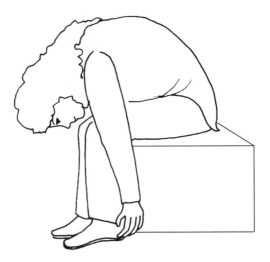

Thoracic-Lumbar Rotators

Sit on the edge of a chair with your back straight and your feet flat on the floor, shoulder width apart. Lock your hands behind your head with your elbows out. Tuck your chin down. Contract your abdominal, oblique, and opposite thoracic-lumbar rotator muscles to rotate your upper body in one direction until you have twisted as far as you can go. When you feel loosened up—after 4 or 5 repetitions in one direction—rotate, hold, and then flex your trunk forward, leading down between your knees toward the ground with your elbow. Return to an upright position. Work one side at a time, completing all repetitions before beginning the opposite side. Hold each stretch 1 to 2 seconds, and then return to the resting position. Do 8 to 10 repetitions. You'll feel this stretch in your lower back and upper hips.

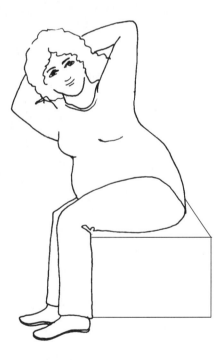

Lateral Trunk Flexors

Sit on the edge of a chair with your back straight and your feet flat on the floor, shoulder width apart for stability. Raise one arm, and place your hand behind your head with the elbow pointed away from your body. Bend at the waist so that the arm that is straight is lowered down the leg of the chair toward the floor, until you feel a little pull in the opposite side of your trunk. Work one side at a time. Hold each stretch 1 to 2 seconds, and then return to the resting position. Do 8 to 10 repetitions. You'll feel this stretch in your sides.

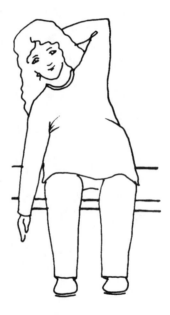

Rhomboid/Rotator Cuff

Sit on the edge of a chair with your back straight and your feet flat on the floor, shoulder width apart for stability. Lift one arm, with your elbow locked, and raise it across your chest toward the opposite shoulder. Use the other hand to give a gentle assist at the elbow at the end of the movement. Keep your torso still. Resist the temptation to "hike" up your shoulder. Work one side at a time. Hold each stretch 1 to 2 seconds, and then return to the resting position. Do 8 to 10 repetitions. You'll feel this stretch in your outer shoulder and upper back.

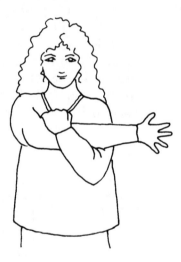

Neck Routine

Sit on the edge of a chair with your back straight and your feet flat on the floor, shoulder width apart for stability. With your hands placed on the back of your head, tuck your chin and roll your head forward until your chin meets your chest. You can gently assist the end of the movement with your hands at the back of your head. Then roll your head straight back, chin up, and gently guide the stretch with your fingertips spread along your jawline. Return to the resting position. Finally, turn your head slightly to one side and then roll it down toward your chest again. You can gently assist the end of the movement with your hands at the back of your head. Return to the resting position. Be certain to keep your shoulders down. Hold each stretch 1 to 2 seconds before returning to the resting position. Do 8 to 10 repetitions of each stretch. You'll feel these stretches in your neck and across your upper back.

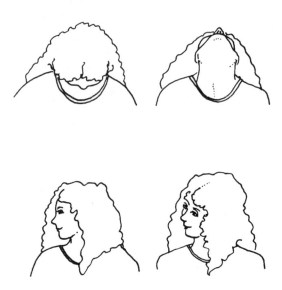

Leg and Foot Cramps

One of the banes of an expectant mother's existence is cramping. We think we can help. The heavier you get, the less you may want to move. Blood flow is reduced, waste products build in muscles, and muscles become flaccid and lethargic. Not good. Keeping a good flex routine will keep your body moving and supple without straining you. Your muscles will be less likely to interpret movement as traumatic and worthy of a good cramp. Blood flow will be increased and metabolic waste will be flushed. You'll get a little workout with every Active-Isolated Stretching session, so your muscles will not atrophy.

Make certain that you are properly fueled and hydrated. Your body is working hard twenty-four hours a day, helping a little person grow. The hydration and nutritional demands for both of you are exceptional. Early in pregnancy, you may experience morning sickness. Nausea and a diminished appetite may severely deplete your stores of water and nutrients. Later in your pregnancy, you may become overly concerned about weight gain and try to cut back on food and drink. Don't do it—unless you are under supervision by your physician or a registered dietitian. Muscles that are not hydrated and fueled will cramp.

How do you relieve a cramp? Simple. To get a muscle to relax and uncramp in record time, you isolate that muscle, identify it as best you can, and contract the *opposite* muscle, assisting the stretch at the end with gentle pressure. Hold for 2 seconds, release, and then do it again in a sort of pumping fashion. For example, a cramp in your calf will relax if you flex your foot up by tensing your shin—the muscle "opposite" your calf. Reach out and pull your foot toward your knee at the end of the stretch. Hold for 2 seconds and release. Relax and then do it again. The principle applies wherever you develop a cramp.

A Final Note

During this very special time in your life, your Active-Isolated Stretching routine can be a valuable tool for maintaining fitness, training safely and gently for labor and delivery, and recovering rapidly after your baby is born. The benefits are more than physical, however. As you learn to isolate and fire specific muscles, you will be learning lessons about your body that will be valuable in the delivery room. Your ability to focus and relax will be greatly enhanced. You'll have more control.

And being focused, relaxed, and in control in the delivery room will help you conserve your energy for the really important task at hand: bringing your child into the world.

Congratulations and best of luck from both of us! (And, if you have a boy, let us know if you name him "James Phillip"?)

Active-Isolated Stretching as We Grow Older

If I had known I was going to live this long, I would have taken better care of myself.

This well-known bumper sticker is intended to make us laugh, but aging is no laughing matter. Doing it well takes hard work—a truth about all things in human performance.

We have been in the fitness business long enough to see a number of our athletes mature from young men and women to "Master" athletes. And we have seen some of our early "Masters" continue to compete, exploding any myths or misconceptions we had about human performance in later years. The truth is that many of the maladies and deficiencies we associate with aging are NOT factors of aging, but effects of becoming sedentary, a condition that is easily mitigated by getting off one's duff. The good news is that it is never too late to begin a fitness program. Indeed, a landmark study on nursing home residents conducted by the U.S. Department of Agriculture Human Nutrition Research Center on Aging at Tufts University and the Hebrew Rehabilitation Center for the Aged revealed that flexibility and strength improved significantly in older people who participated in an exercise program.

Aging appears to coincide with a slow loss of muscle mass—about 1 percent per year after age 30. Muscles are like furnaces that burn fat for energy. As muscle mass diminishes, the body can't burn fat as efficiently, literally becoming less lean and more fat. This combination forms a sort of "vicious cycle": less muscle means more fat means even less muscle which means even more fat which means . . . well, you get the picture. It is called "creeping atrophy" for good reason. It happens slowly, starting as early as our twenties. By the time we notice that

203

body parts are drifting and anatomical peaks and valleys are becoming redistributed, the cycle has a firm hold on us—its victims. Unless checked, the consequences are debilitating and insidious. In the past, we accepted these declines as normal functions of aging, but not any more. Research and experience have demonstrated that we can stay well and healthy in our later years by engaging in a fitness program. In fact, exercise may be the best kept antiaging secret around.

FLEXIBILITY: THE KEY THAT UNLOCKS FITNESS

Fitness is defined as a combination of flexibility, strength, endurance, and cardiovascular health. As we age, flexibility is the key that unlocks all the other components. If you can get your body to move, you can put the other fitness pieces in place, providing that you are medically able to participate.

Active-Isolated Stretching may well be the perfect key. Most of the flex routines can be accomplished from sitting or reclining positions, so the program may be started slowly and gently. This may be particularly important if you're a beginner to the fitness world and are not accustomed to high-energy workouts, or have physical limitations that make it difficult or perilous for you to hang from the rafters or bench press a bar bell or sprint around a track. Stretching requires no special equipment, clothing, or facilities. Its benefit are many. To elongate a muscle (the agonist), you must fire the opposing muscle (the antagonist). The effect is a relaxed, lengthened muscle AND a strengthened muscle. The rhythmic action of your routine pumps blood throughout the area you are stretching. Your heart works a little harder and you breathe a little more deeply—inhaling on the extension phase and exhaling as you relax the position. Indeed, from your first workout, without having to get out of bed, you are isolating and exercising muscles, elongating and strengthening muscles and connective tissues, expanding the ranges of motion on your joints, getting your heart rate up, and enhancing your cardiovascular fitness. Keep it up and soon you will be able to add "endurance" to your list of benefits. The more you do, the more you are able to do. Stronger. Longer. Better. Much better.

We have a client, Martha Harris, who is 88 years old. She came to us at age 86 because "nothing was working right." She was essentially immobile: stooped over and suffering terribly from joint pain. Like most people, when she was in pain, she tended to avoid doing anything that would aggravate the joint. When her knees hurt, she stopped walking. When her neck hurt, she stopped turning her head. When her back hurt, she lay down. When her shoulders hurt, she stopped reaching for things . . . including life. Her world became smaller and smaller until she was bedridden. Her physicians prescribed painkillers, but no one thought of working out as a solution. Everyone assumed that Martha was too old, frail, and fragile to exercise. Except Martha. She read about a study that concluded that exercise programs to increase flexibility had significantly improved range of motion in hips, knees, and ankles in institutionalized elderly subjects. Martha wanted the same—and more—for herself. And she chose us.

We will never forget our first meeting with her. Her range of motion on every joint was as small as we had ever seen. We suggested that she continue to take her daily painkillers so that she would be less likely to respond to discomfort by refusing to move. We worked slowly and carefully, measuring progress by millimeters. She was eager and good-humored, and we were intrigued. Active-Isolated Stretching did its job. The muscles we were stretching eventually began to elongate. The muscles she was firing to relax the elongating muscles began to strengthen. Joints began to unlock. Blood was recruited to areas that had been shut down. The effort from lifting a leg or an arm was intense enough to give her heart and lungs a gentle aerobic-type workout without impact. She became less afraid to move something that hurt. And the hurt started to lessen. The more comfortable Martha became, the more willing she was to move. And the more she moved, the faster she healed. As her muscle mass and her activity level increased, she lost a significant amount of body fat and weight. Today, Martha is up and back in the game of life. Granted, she probably will not run a marathon or pursue a career in ballet, but Martha and her stretch rope are doing just fine.

The Bigger We Are, the Harder We Fall

The purpose of Active-Isolated Stretching is to make certain that you stay flexible for life. The more flexible the body is, the more mobile, balanced, and stable it is. And mobility, balance, and stability—or rather, the lack of them—have been cited among the elderly as the leading factors in falling. When children fall, they generally are quick and resilient enough to mitigate a little tumble. And, they get lots of practice. How do we know? We conducted a highly scientific survey of the Band-Aid™ shelf at our local pharmacy. All the designer models were cartoon characters and super heros. The kid market. One typical scenario? Junior takes a header. Skinned knee. Mom kisses the booboo to make it better. And junior goes on about his business, reminded of the incident only by a Band-Aid™ festooned with 'toons. The scenario is radically different as we mature. The older we get, the harder we fall. First, adults are taller and heavier. Consequently, we have farther to fall and there is more body mass to hit the ground, so the impact is greater. Second, reaction times may be a bit slower, so there is less opportunity to compensate—to make that series of split-second decisions about "catching" oneself. Finally, older people with calcium deficiencies may suffer from bone density loss—osteopenia or osteoporosis—which could make any fall a shattering experience. Research demonstrates conclusively that falling poses a serious health problem for adults over 65 years old, and is the leading cause of accidental death in adults over 75. Once having fallen, a person is statistically more likely to fall again, a fact that older people intuitively have known since before research was invented. After the first fall, an older adult likely will become fearful and cautious, limiting activity. And limited activity means that life starts winding down unnecessarily.

Loosen Up Those Joints

Having joints that are capable of going through their full range of motion allows the muscles and connective tissues to respond to strengthening exercises and decreases the chances of deformity—the gnarling of a joint, which, in the past, has been associated simply with getting older. Unlocking frozen joints recruits blood to the area, bringing in oxygen that nourishes cells and removing waste products that are produced by the locked site, thereby promoting healing. Also, being able to move through a full range means that each joint works as it was intended: strong, stable, balanced, and functional.

One of our clients is a 70-year-old jazz pianist, Ronald Richards, whose hands and fingers were increasingly stiff and sore, preventing him from playing the elaborate pieces he once mastered easily. Striking keys was painful and, worse, unpredictable. He explained, "I reach for a key and there is a 'lag' in my timing. My brain knows what to do, but my hands can't respond fast enough." Throughout his career, he had been well known for his ability to play music so complicated and fast-paced that his hands were virtual blurs on the keyboard. But a lifetime of sitting at the piano and pounding the ivories apparently had taken their toll. The tips of his fingers were flexed painfully at the first joints,

206

locked into little crooks. He was forced to modify his key strikes: hitting a key with the pad of a finger was replaced by thumping it with the tip. His hands, wrists, elbows, and shoulders strained from the effort. The trauma to each joint escalated with every note.

Ronald stoically had accepted his fate as the inevitable course of aging, and slowly had evolved a number of compensations: playing more slowly, playing less frequently, playing only in the afternoon or evening after he had warmed up during the day, playing less elaborate pieces . . . until the day came when he could no longer play at all. And for a musician, this was an inconceivable conclusion to a satisfying career. Frustrated, he visited our clinic to see whether we could do anything to reverse the lockup. Smart man. There was a lot we could do to help. At our first session, we convinced him that he was a whole person who deserved a healthy body. It was important to unlock his entire body, so we worked with him to increase the range of motion in his hands, wrists, elbows, shoulders, neck, back, hip, and trunk. Then we concentrated on his fingers. Because he was a pianist, his fingers were strong, but the muscles had become imbalanced as each strained to compensate or became atrophied from disuse. Slowly, as we gently worked, his fingers began to unlock. Blood, carrying healing oxygen, was recruited to each joint. Muscles that were tight, elongated. Muscles that were atrophied, fired. The recovery process had begun, and Ronald was thrilled. Today, he is back to playing concerts and enjoying a resurgence in his career . . . and his health.

Sleep Like a Baby

As we age, we need less sleep. We would like to think that what we lack in quantity of sleep could be made up in quality, but this tends to be untrue. For many older people, sleep isn't short and sweet. It's short and problematic. One theory is that an older person slows down physically and a sedentary lifestyle doesn't tire the body out. Although the person might be mentally and emotionally exhausted, the body—still raring to go—stages a mutiny at bedtime, punishing its owner with a seemingly endless night of tossing and turning. Additionally, it may be difficult to fall asleep and stay asleep when the body is uncomfortable, wracked by joint pain and unable to relax.

Researchers tell us that exercise enhances a good night's sleep. We agree. Interestingly, these same reports advise us to refrain from exercising late at night within a couple of hours of bedtime, suggesting that exercise can overstimulate us and make it difficult to fall asleep. We disagree. Maybe we would become overstimulated if we attended an aerobic dance class just before bedtime, but Active-Isolated Stretching gives us a good workout and relaxes us at the same time. (The only problem is keeping straight faces as we attempt to explain eight-foot ropes at our bedsides.) Many of our older clients—and we ourselves—work out in bed right before we fall asleep, to ensure a good night's sleep. And, in the morning, we roll out of bed without grunting and groaning. Our older clients report that they awaken without stiffness.

KEEPING YOUR BONES STRONG

One of the maladies that seems to typify the fragility of an elderly person is falling and breaking a hip. We have a news flash for you. More often than you could imagine, first the hip breaks and THEN the person falls. Osteoporosis is demineralization of bone that causes it to weaken and makes it unable to withstand even the slightest trauma or to support minimal weight. The pelvis, which serves as the foundation for both the upper and lower body, takes a lot of stress as it stabilizes the body for movement. When the pelvis is weakened and thinned from osteoporosis, it may be unable to hold up and may give way in a searing fracture, dropping its owner to the ground. Indeed, osteoporosis is the reason we have the term "little old lady." The "little" comes from the sad fact that many women literally shrink as their bone masses decrease and they suffer from vertebral fractures that diminish their height. This collapse of spine forms the "Dowager's Hump" at the base of the neck, when the back can no longer support the weight of the head and the neck drops forward. Abdominal and thoracic organs get repositioned as the spine slowly collapses behind them and the rib cage closes in. Anatomically, very little will work properly past this point. The pain is described as being agonizing and relentless. Men and women, young and old, are susceptible to osteopenia (the precursor) and osteoporosis, but postmenopausal women may be more at risk.

Osteoporosis or osteopenia are easily diagnosed with a bone scan—a safe and painless procedure that gives a person and his or her physician an accurate reading of bone density. The physician may scan the entire body or select a small but representative part of the body, such as the hip or wrist, for a miniscan.

The good news is that osteoporosis is preventable with good healthcare. Once detected, it may be slowed or partially reversed. Physicians recommend that calcium supplements be added to the diet and exercise be made part of life. A study from the Washington University School of Medicine in St. Louis has determined that it is important to exercise three times a week for 30 minutes each session, for strength and aerobic conditioning. Exercising women in the study gained 6.2 percent more bone mass in just two years; their sedentary counterparts continued to lose bone mass.

Posture Is More Than Looking Good

Eighty percent of all older adults complain at some point of low back pain. How often have you heard "I've got a bad back"—or said it yourself? The source of low back pain is rarely the lower back. Pain comes from weakened abdominal muscles that no longer allow an older person to support proper carriage. To prove the point to yourself, stand up straight and thrust your lower abdomen out, exaggerating the "paunch" of a weakened midline. Notice that your lower back follows forward and your hips rock forward to form a sort of front-to-back "S"-curve. Your waist disappears. Your head thrusts forward. Your internal organs shift. And your breathing becomes shallow. When so many things shift and change, your body enters into a series of compensations to adjust to the new posture. Your back, from the base of your skull to the flair of your pelvis, strains against this forward pull to hold you erect. And something—probably your back—is guaranteed to give. A strong abdomen will help keep your body in line.

Another leading cause of "bad backs" is lack of flexibility. One of the sayings in Tai Chi is: "You are as young as your spine is flexible." Keeping your spine supple allows you to move freely and to hold your body in perfect form. You will have a hedge on injury. Your back "gives" when you reach for something or move suddenly.

Flexibility Is Smart

Not only is Active-Isolated Stretching smart for your body, but studies have shown that exercise can increase your mental functioning as well by increasing the blood flow to your brain. Test scores are better than those of nonexercising people and are improved when a person starts to exercise. Additionally, response times are quicker.

Fit People Live Longer and Better

C. Everett Koop, M.D., former Surgeon General of the United States, has linked five of the top ten "killers" in the U.S. to lifestyle, specifically obesity. The deadly five are heart disease, some forms of cancer, diabetes, stroke, and atherosclerosis. He also blamed obesity for osteoarthritis, gout, and a number of mental health problems. Anything that is related to lifestyle—including obesity—is YOUR personal responsibility. These disorders can be prevented or, once diagnosed, mitigated with a little effort on your part at any age. MOVE! The reward? Good health.

It seems that good health begets good health. Studies have demonstrated that physically fit people have healthier immune systems than non-exercising people, and are better able to ward off bacteria, yeast, and some viruses with elevated levels of immunoglobulin.

In addition to good health, one of the real advantages of your fitness program is self-esteem. With every inch you lose from your waist, every degree you gain in range of motion, every extra pound you lift, or every extra foot you walk, you will feel better about yourself. You owe it to yourself to organize a personal fitness program centered around a base of flexibility. We absolutely guarantee that you will be happier and more relaxed, live longer, and function better throughout your life. In the words of Rabbi Ben Ezra (1864),

> Grow old along with me!
> The best is yet to be,
> The last of life, for which the first was made . . .

Body Language: Understanding What Your Body Is Saying

We once had an athlete-client who ignored clear signals—warning signs—from her body until it broke down with a serious injury right before an important international competition. We were incredulous. This injury should have been no surprise. When we discussed the events that led to the injury, we all agreed that she should have known it was coming. We asked her, "Don't you listen to your body?" She replied, "I hear it. I guess I just don't know what it says."

She is not alone. Over the years, a number of people in our care have described "strange" sounds. More than once, a client has grabbed one of us by the head and pressed a Wharton ear to a joint with the stern order to "Listen!" We're used to it. When we listen, we can interpret. Sometimes, the message your body sends is not an audible sound, but a sound you can feel with your fingers. Sometimes the message has no sound and no vibration—it's more of a "feeling." Or, it's something you can see on the surface. No matter how you receive the message, you need to be able to interpret it. To aid your interpretation, we compiled a vocabulary list. We call it "Body Language."

SIGNALS YOU CAN FEEL

Aching   This is dull, low-level, persistent pain. Usually you feel aching when your body is at rest, and it feels better when you get moving and the area is warmed up. Aching generally means that a muscle, ligament, or tendon is contracted, or you could have a nerve impingement. Aching is a signal that something more acute or serious is just around the corner. Resist the common temptation to ignore your aches. Pay attention to them.

Asleep (More extreme than tingling.) Blood flow is constricted or a nerve is impinged, shutting down neurological transmissions to that area. If it is a fleeting condition, it is no problem. If it recurs or lasts more than a few minutes, you need to seek medical attention.

Cold Muscles could be so contracted that they have lost circulation, usually in extremities such as feet and hands. You need to get moving. Open the area up with Active-Isolated Stretching to restore range of motion and blood flow.

Cramping A muscle is severely contracted. Common causes are dehydration, overuse, or inactivity. Relax the muscle by firing the opposite muscle and stretching the cramped one.

Fatigue This is the manifestation of the body's inability to continue to function. It could be general fatigue, a symptom of poor nutrition or a medical condition, or, when localized, it could be overuse. If you are a very active person who gets tired, you need to recover: get rest, nutrition, and hydration, and increase your flexibility. If rest doesn't relieve the fatigue, see a healthcare professional. If it is localized and you can't tie the fatigue to a specific cause, see a healthcare professional.

Feeling faint Blood supply to your brain is inadequate. This could have a number of causes, which you will figure out later. Your immediate attention should be focused on maintaining consciousness and avoiding hitting the ground. Lie down and elevate your feet. Or, sit down and put your head between your knees. If you can't figure out what caused it or if it recurs, seek medical attention.

Flipping	A muscle, tendon, or ligament may slip over a boney prominence or a hypermobile joint. If there is no pain, don't worry. If there is pain, you need to be medically evaluated to determine whether nature's design has a flaw or you have become so tight in a joint that you are literally pulling out of alignment, causing the flip. Loosen up the joint with flexibility and strength.
Grinding	This is the sound of bone on bone, or particles floating in fluid, or a muscle, tendon, or ligament sliding over bone. If there is no pain, don't worry. If there is pain, you need to be medically evaluated to determine whether nature's design has a flaw or you have become so tight in a joint that you are literally pulling out of alignment, causing the grind. Loosen up the joint with flexibility and strength.
Hot	You may have torn a muscle microscopically, or the heat could result from metabolic waste or lactic acid buildup after intense activity. Infection or a trauma with swelling is also possible. Any body part that feels hot requires your attention.
Itching	This happens to muscles that are unaccustomed to working hard and being pumped full of blood. It subsides after the muscles cool down. No problem, unless you see a rash.
Knotty	Individual muscle fibers have torn and realigned randomly in little clumps. You can self-massage them to break them up and help them realign. Then you need to initiate a strength and flexibility program.
Lack of coordination	The body is unable to receive neurological signals and/or react to signals. This could be caused by genetics, dehydration, exhaustion, vascular accidents, or neurological disorders. If the onset of lack of coordination is sudden, you need to seek medical attention immediately.
Lumpy	A muscle is weak. There are inconsistencies in the muscle fibers. You need a strength and flexibility program. (We see this most frequently in the lower back, at the top of the pelvis.)

Mushy	A muscle is weak and has no integrity. You need a strength and flexibility program. (We see this most frequently on the inside of the top of the knee where the inner quad attaches to and stabilizes the knee.)
Pain	Pain is a wonderful thing. It is the clearest, most articulate communication your body can send. It means, "Something is wrong!" The stronger the signal, the louder the message. Avoid the temptation to ignore the signal or mask it with painkillers before you know for certain what the source of the pain is. Pay attention.
Quivering	The muscle has "shorted out" and is experiencing rapid, continuous firing. Quivering is frequently the result of intense fatigue; it could also be an early warning sign of cramp. Relieve the tension with Active-Isolated Stretching, massage the area with ice, and then take a little rest. Make certain that you are hydrated.
Reverberation	This is aftershock of a released adhesion or flipping. No problem.
Rip	When you hear a rip, it could be something tearing. If it is accompanied by pain, have it evaluated immediately; connective tissue or fascia around the muscle could be stretching.
Shock	A nerve is suddenly impinged by a muscle passing over or under it, or pressing against it. This is generally no problem. If it recurs, you need to isolate the muscle and unlock the tension in the impinged area. Restore flexibility and range of motion.
Side stitch	Your diaphragm muscles cramp or contract under your rib cage. It happens when you breathe too hard and your diaphragm has to work hard to keep up with the expanding and contracting of your lungs. Some people have problems when they eat or drink too heavily before they work out. No problem. Relieve it by taking slow, deep, full breaths. Lift your arms up over your head (yes, you can do this while you're running) and extend them behind your head as far as you can get them. This will open up your chest and allow you to bring in more oxygen.

Spasm	The muscle is in contraction. This is a cramp, but it is sometimes distinguished by "waves" of contraction rather than the "death grip" characterized by a cramp. Immediately fire the opposite muscle and gently stretch out the spasming muscle with an assist at the end of the stretch. This will relax the muscle that is in spasm.
Tenderness	Pain is your body's clear signal that something is damaged and needs protection or attention. Tenderness is low-level pain.
Tension	The muscle is irritated, causing constriction of blood flow. The source could be physical or emotional. Tension is generally no problem, but it can lead to damaging compensation patterns in the musculoskeletal system over time. Relax.
Throbbing	The area is constricted and sensitive, and you can feel the blood flow as a "pulse." If the throbbing is accompanied by swelling (and it generally is), you need to pay attention.
Tingling	Blood flow is constricted or a nerve has been impinged and is interfering with neurological transmissions to that area. Tingling has the potential to shut the whole area down. You need to find the source of impingement and alleviate it. First, try unlocking with Active-Isolated Stretching. If that doesn't work, seek medical attention.

SIGNALS YOU CAN HEAR

Clicking	A bone could be a little bit out of joint, caused possibly by tight muscles pulling the joint out of alignment. This is usually not a big problem and Active-Isolated Stretching can help.
Creaking	Muscles, tendons, and ligaments are tight. Loosen up. There may not be enough fluid in a joint, so it is not well lubricated. If creaking is accompanied by pain, seek medical attention.

Crunching	Usually found in the neck, hands, and feet, calcification forms around the joints at the muscle attachments. Crunches are, in themselves, not a problem, but they are early warning signs that you need to keep those joints moving and maintain good joint range of motion.
Gristing	A tight muscle pulls at the joint and compresses the bones on either side of the joint. This could be the sound of irregularities of the articular cartilage, which could eventually lead to irritation.
Loud pop	If a pop happens in trauma, it could mean a muscle tear or detachment, and requires your immediate attention. If it's followed by minor swelling, it could be a ligament pull, tear, or detachment. If the pop is followed by major swelling, it could be a muscle.
Pop	An adhesion—something once torn or traumatized and stuck to bone—may be suddenly released. No problem. Your body just did you a favor. Or, this could be a bone breaking. Big problem: Dial 911. It could also be a hamstring pull, requiring medical attention, or a musculoskeletal adjustment, as when your back pops out of subluxation. Rule of thumb: If the pop hurts, check it out.
Snap	This could be an adhesion giving way—something once torn or traumatized and stuck to bone is suddenly released. It could also be a bone fracturing, a sprain, or a tendon tearing loose. If the snap is accompanied by pain, or if you can't bear weight on that joint, check it out with a healthcare professional.

SIGNALS YOU CAN SEE

Bruising	This is a leakage of blood from a trauma such as an external blow or an internal tear. Pay attention.
Redness	Blood has rushed to the surface after hard exercise or following trauma. If it is exercise induced, it will go

away when you cool down. If it is from trauma and is accompanied by pain or doesn't go away, pay attention.

Swelling   Fluid may have accumulated when your body has not been able to flush sufficiently. This could also be an infection; a symptom of a trauma or injury, where the body rushes to the site with fluid for protection and flushing out waste material; or an accumulation of blood deep in the muscle. You need to pay attention to this.

Stretching or Surgery?

Injury. It might as well be a four-letter word. It gets the same reaction. It is the dreaded "shutdown" that every athlete fears and despises. At best, an injury will take all the fun out of a workout. At worst, it can mean the end of an athlete's career. Injury can happen slowly, sneaking up on someone who isn't paying attention to all the body's warning signs. Or, it can happen quickly, in an unexpected collision or fall on the playing field. Injury can happen while playing your sport or two hours after, when you are headed home. It is part and parcel of being an athlete . . . and a human being. To sum up injury: anything can happen anytime and anywhere.

CHOOSING THE ROPE OR THE KNIFE

Occasionally, your body breaks down to such an extent that someone will suggest surgery to you. Indeed, surgical intervention is the only way to repair many injuries or conditions, but we thought you might enjoy knowing that some injuries and conditions can be mitigated with Active-Isolated Stretching BEFORE they become so serious that a surgeon has to be involved.

If you experience such an injury or medical condition, consult your physician and pay close attention to the advice you are given. But, if you are able, reach for your stretch rope before he or she reaches for the knife. Generally, a sports medicine expert will encourage you to try nonsurgical procedures before resorting to the operating room. Again, consult your physician.

Injuries and Conditions That May Respond Well to Active-Isolated Stretching

Injury 1. Achilles Tendon Contracture (Shortening)

The Achilles tendon—the cord that runs from the back of the heel to the calf—shortens, causing an inability to dorsiflex the ankle. To explain, if the athlete stands flat on the ground, he or she cannot pivot the foot up with the heel on the ground. The foot eventually weakens, causing pain in the midfoot, the calf, and along the longitudinal arch. Women who wear high-heeled shoes may be particularly vulnerable. Surgery lengthens the tendon.

In 1991, American Dennis Mitchell, who later won the Olympic gold medal as a member of the 4 × 100 meters relay team at Barcelona, competed in a meet in Sicily at the end of the European track and field season. He was running spectacularly when suddenly he pulled up, grabbing the back of his foot. We carried him from the track, immediately packed him in ice to ease the pain and swelling, and evaluated the injury. Unquestionably, we thought it was his Achilles tendon. This was the season before the Olympic Games, and this was the injury we didn't want. Jim Wharton and Dennis flew straight back to Gainesville, Florida, where Dennis trained. They met with Dr. Karl Weingarten, who ordered an MRI (magnetic resonance imaging) scan. It confirmed our suspicions. Dennis indeed had acute Achilles tendinitis—microtears in the tendon. We went right to work. His coach was able to delay his return to practice for a month while we launched an intensive rehabilitation program that involved icing, Active-Isolated Stretching, and strength workouts. One month later, Dr. Weingarten evaluated our progress with a second MRI. Healing was well underway. In 1992, Dennis won the U.S. Track and Field Trials in the 100 meters and made the U.S. Olympic team. At the Olympic Games in Barcelona, he won the bronze medal in 100 meters (he was the only American medalist in that event. He even beat Carl Lewis!). And he won the gold in the 4 × 100 relay. Not bad for a guy we had to carry off the track a few short months before.

To avoid Achilles tendon contracture, concentrate your flexibility work on Lower Legs, Ankles, and Feet (Active-Isolated Stretches 47–59).

Injury 2. Hallux Valgus (Bunions)

The big toe is angled over or under the toe next to it, forming a "lump" at the side of the juncture where the big toe meets the body of the foot. The pressure on this angle causes the bursa of the joint to become inflamed and infected. Eventually, the bones deform. In compensating, the foot distributes extra pressure on the head of the first toe, so the bone grows bigger to handle the weight. The gait is adjusted to accommodate a changing distribution of pressure and weight. The condition may be genetically linked and may be exacerbated by wearing shoes that are too tight. Surgery trims the bunion and straightens the toes.

In 1988, runner Lynn Nelson was the U.S. Olympic Trials champion in the 10,000 meters, but that splendid performance was followed by a season of injury. Like many runners, her feet took a terrible pounding and there was a price to pay. Tendons in her feet were shortened, and her feet were being pulled out of alignment. Painful bunions threw her footstrikes off. Her body was doing the best it could with functional compensations to make up for the imbalances, but, frankly, things were coming unglued for her. At first, there were little injuries. And then bigger ones. A brilliant career for a wonderful, talented, hardworking athlete was coming to an end. Until she put Active-Isolated Stretching into her program. The turnaround didn't happen overnight, but it did happen. She qualified for the U.S. Olympic Trials for the marathon at the 1996 Summer Games in Atlanta.

To avoid hallus valgus, concentrate your flexibility work on Lower Legs, Ankles, and Feet (Active-Isolated Stretches 47–59).

Injury 3.   Hammer Toes

This is a condition that causes the toes to curl down into "claws." It is a double deformity: an extension deformity of the first "knuckle" of the toe (pointing it up) and a flexion deformity of the other "knuckles" (pointing them down). It may be caused by poorly fitting shoes or shortened tendons and muscles in the top of the foot, which draw the toes up. Because the toes can't function properly, foot movement is impeded. The body must engage a series of compensations to make up for weakness and deformity. Surgery straightens the toes.

In 1992, U.S. National Champion (1991) runner John Trautman won the U.S. Olympic Trials in New Orleans in the 5,000 meters. And he did it with painful nerve impingement caused by hammer toes. Unfortunately, the miles and the poundings took their toll and he ended up severely injured. He had surgery in Houston to release his toes and relieve the impingements, but, like all driven runners, he "forgot" to rehabilitate before he hit the track again. His body cooperated at first. It initiated a series of clever compensations to balance feet that were weakened and dynamics that were unfamiliar. But when his body realized that John intended to run it into the ground, it rebelled by tightening up and then delivering a punishing pelvic stress fracture. Everyone close to him—including his family—said, "Hang up your running shoes. It's time for you to look for a job." But running was at the heart of John Trautman. Together, we three designed a rehab program for him, centered around Active-Isolated Stretching and strength workouts. His recovery was slow. He had to work hard—and still does. We are proud to report that he did NOT hang up his shoes and get a job. Instead, he represented the United States in the World Cross Country Championships that year.

To avoid hammer toes, concentrate your flexibility work on Lower Legs, Ankles, and Feet (Active-Isolated Stretches 47–59).

Injury 4. Chronic Low Back Pain

One of the most common complaints among all people is low back pain—particularly in the lower lumbar region and the sacrum (across the back of the pelvis). It can be caused by many things, but frequently can be traced to injury, weakness, intervertebral disk abnormality, disease, or abnormal function somewhere else in the body. Experience tells us to suspect weak abdominal muscles. Surgery fuses the spine to the pelvis to stabilize the area and shore up weakness.

Poland's Wanda Panfil is one of the greatest marathon runners in the world, and one of the nicest people. She has won the Boston Marathon, the New York City Marathon, and the World Championships. But marathon training and running are brutal, and Wanda has to balance that fine line between "enough miles" and "too many miles." At one point in her career, she made the mistake of crossing that line, and the consequences were insidious. She parlayed a chronic low back pain into a serious hip injury that launched her on a quest for solutions: surgery and cortisone shots and rehabilitation protocols that ran the gamut. Everything worked . . . for a little while. But the setbacks became more frequent and more severe until she was nearly shut down. She flew to New York, where we worked intensively for three days with Active-Isolated Stretching. At the end of three days, she headed out our front door for a five-mile test jog and returned to the clinic a believer. We sent her back to her home in Mexico City with a stretch rope and our best wishes. She is on the comeback trail.

To avoid chronic low back pain, concentrate your flexibility work on Upper Legs, Hip, and Trunk (Active-Isolated Stretches 1–17).

Injury 5. Radio-humeral Bursitis (Tennis Elbow)

Tennis elbow is an overuse injury. It may be caused by the wrist's being continuously turned to the outside against resistance—such as when using a screwdriver—or by turning the wrist to the inside when the arm is explosively extended—such as when executing a driving backhand in a tennis game. The pain, usually on the outside of the arm, can be debilitating. The wrist weakens; specifically, it is increasingly unable to "cock" up, as in the gesture made for "Stop!" Surgery may include manipulation under anesthetic, curettement, and (fortunately, rarely) excision.

Brooke Herman is a nationally ranked junior player who lives in New York. She is also a bright, sprightly teenager with a tennis career in her pocket and the world at her feet. And an aching arm that threatened all that. Tennis elbow can be a problem for people of all ages, and Brooke proves it. Typically, when the injured arm starts to weaken, the body does its best to find other ways to do its job. The result? A series of imbalances in other areas. Eventually, the athlete has the original injury with compounded interest. Such was the case with Brooke. She started out with an irritation and it escalated into other problems. When she was referred to us by Aaron Mattes, we started a program of Active-Isolated Stretching and strengthening. She worked hard and continues to do so. There are no magic answers, but the work is worth the effort. Broke has a full college scholarship and a promising future in tennis.

To avoid tennis elbow, concentrate your flexibility work on Arms, Elbows, Wrists, and Hands (Active-Isolated Stretches 35–46).

Injury 6. Tendinitis

Tendinitis is an inflammation of a tendon—the connector between muscle and bone. It may be caused by degeneration or repeated trauma such as overuse. Most frequently at risk are the shoulder capsule, the outside of the forearm (flexor carpi ulnaris), the finger (flexor digitorum), the hip capsule, the back of the thigh (hamstrings), and the cord that runs from the back of the heel to the calf (Achilles tendon). Surgery may include cutting the sheath around the tendon, freeing it.

Anthony Nesty, of Surinam, is the greatest 100-meters butterfly swimmer who ever lived. He holds the Olympic record and has won every major championship in the world. We met in 1989 in Gainesville,

Florida, when he came to us with a frozen shoulder, the result of tendinitis so severe that it literally shut him down. He was in terrible pain. His hand and fingers were numb. And worse, he had been out of the pool for seven days. The pressure was really on him. A competition was coming up within the month: a rematch with Matt Biondi, the first after the Olympic Games, where the media had questioned Anthony's win over Biondi as a fluke. Winning a second time was important to Anthony. There was something to prove. And some disbelievers to convert. Seldom has an athlete been so motivated. Anthony agreed to a total program. He would work out in the pool and then come to the clinic, where Phil would run with him. Then we would put him through an entire Active-Isolated Stretching routine with special emphasis on the frozen shoulder. He would go to class at the University of Florida, take a nap, swim, and then come back to the clinic to lift weights. He worked as hard as anyone we had ever seen. From the daily regimen, his shoulder unlocked and his body became more balanced and finely tuned. In two weeks, he was back into full training. In four weeks, Anthony Nesty defeated Matt Biondi a second time. To this day, Anthony travels with his stretch rope.

To avoid tendinitis, concentrate your flexibility work on applicable Active-Isolated Stretches.

Injury 7.   Osteoarthritis

Arthritis, an inflammation of joints, may come on quickly or progressively. Symptoms may include pain, swelling, stiffness, depression and fatigue, and deformities (gnarling). Surgery is used to remove or replace joints, or to remove degenerated tissue from the joints.

Eva Engdahl-Tegestam is a professional jazz pianist from Sweden whom we met in New York City in the spring of 1995. A lifetime of playing had taken its toll on her hands. She had been diagnosed with arthritis. Her knuckles were swollen and bent. She was losing strength and endurance. The range of motion on each finger was dwindling. And she was in pain. Playing her piano was not as much fun as it once had been. It didn't take more than a single session of Active-Isolated Stretching to start things back the other way. We worked gently on her arms, wrists, hands, and fingers to make small gains in ranges of motion and increase blood flow to each joint. Was it helping? Her broad smile let us know that we were succeeding. "My hands feel more alive. Warmer. Easier to move," she reported. We were privileged to visit Eva in a recording studio that week, where she was in the process of exhausting her much younger backup musicians. Her music was magic. And she was brilliant.

To avoid arthritis, concentrate your flexibility work on applicable Active-Isolated Stretches.

Injury 8.   Carpal Tunnel Syndrome

Recently described as "epidemic" among keyboard users, carpal tunnel syndrome is a classic overuse injury. Keyboards are not the only culprits. Other specific repetitive movements, such as guitar playing, can cause the syndrome. It involves nerve entrapment in the wrist and causes functional impairment such as numbness and weakness, degeneration of muscle, and severe, chronic pain. Indeed, this syndrome is so notorious that it has spawned an industry of its own: braces, cushioning products, and ergonomically friendly work stations and equipment. Surgery releases the carpal tunnel and unblocks the nerve.

George Wandenius is a great guitar player. He has played with Blood, Sweat, and Tears, Steely Dan, and the Saturday Night Live Band. He came to us in pain, unable to extend his "picking" arm. He was experiencing numbness and weakness. His endurance was on the decline. And he couldn't move fast enough to hit a note on time. About to go into a studio to cut an album and then go out on tour, he had a lot of concern about his ability to perform. He came to us for help. (Not only is he a great musician, but he is smart!) From thirty years of playing guitar, George was suffering from a classic overuse injury: carpal tunnel syndrome. We worked from his shoulders to his fingertips with Active-Isolated Stretching. After one session, he could extend his arm almost fully. After several sessions, we all three decided that his next album was going to be a piece of cake and the tour was no problem (as long as he took a stretch rope with him and did his homework faithfully!).

To avoid carpal tunnel syndrome, concentrate your flexibility work on Arms, Elbows, Wrists, and Hands (Active-Isolated Stretches 35–46).

Injury 9.   Scoliosis (Curvature of the Spine)

Scoliosis is an imbalance that causes a C-shaped curvature of the back. Although it may be congenital, it is commonly the result of a compensation by the body to bring itself back into balance when one side of the back is weaker than the other. Surgery is used to implant rods down either side of the spine to brace it into a straightened, upright position.

In high school, Phil Wharton (WHO!?!) was an up-and-coming runner who averaged 35 miles of running per week and took his summers off to rest and recover from the poundings endured during the school year. All was well. Then he went to college and ramped up his running to 80 miles per week. Suddenly, things started going wrong. He began to experience severe back pain that nothing seemed to relieve. Not massage. Not rest. Not rolfing. Not chiropractors. Not medications. The team physicians at the University of Florida diagnosed Phil with scoliosis—curvature of the spine—and suggested implanting rods in his spine to straighten it. They also informed him that if he didn't stop running he could suffer even more debilitating symptoms—up to nerve damage and paralysis. Despairing, and looking for a nonsurgical solution, Phil found Aaron Mattes in Sarasota, Florida, and traveled down the coast to meet with him. Aaron did a muscle-by-muscle evaluation of Phil's body, pointing out areas that were weak and imbalanced. He also told Phil that he thought the scoliosis had nothing to do with the spine. It had everything to do with Phil's being out of balance on one side and drawing his spine into curvature. Aaron told him that he thought he could help. And he did. After one session with Aaron, Phil felt relief. Phil worked with Active-Isolated Stretching and strengthening exercises five hours a day for one year. Once a week, he would travel to Sarasota to Aaron's clinic. During the week, he worked on his own. His spine straightened and his pain disappeared. He returned to running—100 miles per week. Not only did Phil find a solution to his problem, but eventually became a student of Aaron Mattes. And the rest is history. Happily.

To avoid scoliosis, concentrate your flexibility work on Upper Legs, Hip, and Trunk (Active-Isolated Stretches 1–17).

Injury 10. Plantar Fasciitis

This is an inflammation of the plantar fascia—the fibrous connector that runs from the heel to the heads of the metatarsal bones. When the pressure from the heel side is too great, the irritation may form a heel spur—a ridge of bone within the substance of the muscle (flexor digitorum brevis). The symptoms are morning stiffness in the foot and extreme pain. Occasionally, the plantar fascia may rupture following multiple cortisone shots and activity. Surgery releases the medial attachment of the plantar fascia from the inside of the heel bone. The heelspur may be removed.

Jim Wharton (WHO!?!) is a talented recreational runner who logs about 30 to 40 miles a week. Running, he says, gives him joy and helps keep him in great shape for a profession that makes serious demands on his body. Because running is such an important part of his life, he takes care to wear the proper running shoes. When a pair is showing a little wear, they are lovingly retired and replaced. The man, after all, is a fitness professional and, as such, knows how to take such good care of his feet. This is why it is so shocking that Jim Wharton fell in love with a pair of flashy new boots that weren't particularly comfortable, but looked spectacular. He slid them on and headed out for a day in the streets of New York City, walking for miles on concrete sidewalks. Until he finally noticed that he was limping. He took a cab home and took the boots off. The next morning, when he flung himself over the side of his bed, he couldn't put weight on his feet. He had strained the plantar fascia under each foot. The pain was searing. And running was out of the question. It seemed that the master had a lesson to learn. So he iced and added an intensive Active-Isolated Stretching program to his regular one. He put the boots in the back of the closet, where they still look spectacular. Jim healed. And was humbled.

To avoid plantar fasciitis, concentrate your flexibility work on Lower Legs, Ankles, and Feet (Active-Isolated Stretches 47–59).

Forms to Photocopy

PERSONAL ACTIVE-ISOLATED STRETCHING PROGRAM

ZONE 1
Upper Legs, Hips and Trunk
(The Foundation)

1. Single Leg Pelvic Tilt
2. Double Leg Pelvic Tilt
3. Bent Leg Hamstrings
4. Straight Leg Hamstrings
5. Hip Adductors
6. Hip Abductors
7. Psoas
8. Quadriceps
9. Gluteals
10. Trunk Rotators
11. Piriformis
12. Hip External Rotators
13. Hip Internal Rotators
14. Medial Hip Rotators
15. Trunk Extensors
16. Thoracic-Lumbar Rotators
17. Lateral Trunk Flexors

Date _____

NOTES

PERSONAL ACTIVE-ISOLATED STRETCHING PROGRAM

ZONE 2
Shoulders

18. Shoulder Circumduction
19. Pectoralis Major
20. Anterior Deltoid
21. Shoulder Internal Rotators
22. Shoulder External Rotators
23. Rhomboid/Rotator Cuff
24. Trapezius/Rotator Cuff
25. Forward Elev of Shoulder
26. Sideways Elev of Shoulder
27. Posterior Hand Clasp

NOTES

Date _____

PERSONAL ACTIVE-ISOLATED STRETCHING PROGRAM

ZONE 3
Neck

28. Neck Semi-Circumduction
29. Neck Extensors
30. Neck Flexors
31. Neck Lateral Flexors
32. Neck Rotators
33. Neck Oblique Extensors
34. Neck Oblique Flexors

NOTES

Date _____

PERSONAL ACTIVE-ISOLATED STRETCHING PROGRAM

ZONE 4
Arms, Elbows, Wrists, and Hands

	NOTES
35. Elbow Flexors	
36. Biceps	
37. Triceps	
38. Radio-Ulnar Supinators	
39. Radio-Ulnar Pronators	
40. Wrist Flexors—Palms Down	
41. Wrist Flexors—Palms Up	
42. Wrist Extensors	
43. Finger Flexors	
44. Finger Extensors	
45. Straight Finger Rotation	
46. Finger Webbing/Adductor	

Date _____

PERSONAL ACTIVE-ISOLATED STRETCHING PROGRAM

ZONE 5
Lower Legs, Ankles, and Feet

47. Soleus
48. Achilles Tendon
49. Gastrocnemius
50. Tibialis Anterior
51. Ankle Evertors
52. Ankle Invertors
53. Foot Pronators
54. Foot Supinators
55. Metatarsal Arch
56. Toe Extensors
57. Toe Flexors
58. Big Toe Adductor
59. Toe Webbing

NOTES

Date _____

RANGE OF MOTION EVALUATION
ZONE 1
Upper Legs, Hips and Trunk
(The Foundation)

		Degree of Range of Motion	Red	Yellow	Green	Blue
					Range—Check (✔) One	
1. Single Leg Pelvic Tilt	Right					
	Left					
2. Double Leg Pelvic Tilt						
3. Bent Leg Hamstrings	Right					
	Left					
4. Straight Leg Hamstrings	Right					
	Left					
5. Hip Adductors	Right					
	Left					
6. Hip Abductors	Right					
	Left					
7. Psoas	Right					
	Left					
8. Quadriceps	Right					
	Left					
9. Gluteals						
10. Trunk Rotators	Right					
	Left					
11. Piriformis	Right					
	Left					
12. Hip External Rotators	Right					
	Left					
13. Hip Internal Rotators	Right					
	Left					
14. Medial Hip Rotators	Right					
	Left					
15. Trunk Extensors						
16. Thoracic-Lumbar Rotators						
Rotation	Right					
	Left					
Flexion	Right					
	Left					
17. Lateral Trunk Flexors	Right					
	Left					

Date _____

RANGE OF MOTION EVALUATION
ZONE 2
Shoulders

Range—Check (✔) One

	Degree of Range of Motion	Red	Yellow	Green	Blue
18. Shoulder Circumduction	**No Range**				
19. Pectoralis Major Right					
Left					
20. Anterior Deltoid Right					
Left					
21. Shoulder Internal Rotators Right					
Left					
22. Shoulder External Rotators Right					
Left					
23. Rhomboid/Rotator Cuff Right					
Left					
24. Trapezius/Rotator Cuff Right					
Left					
25. Forward Elev of Shoulder Right					
Left					
26. Sideways Elev of Shoulder Right					
Left					
27. Posterior Hand Clasp Right					
Left					

Date _____

RANGE OF MOTION EVALUATION

ZONE 3
Neck

	Degree of Range of Motion	Red	Yellow	Green	Blue
28. Neck Semi-Circumduction					
29. Neck Extensors					
30. Neck Flexors Right					
Left					
31. Neck Lateral Flexors Right					
Left					
32. Neck Rotators Right					
Left					
33. Neck Oblique Extensors Right					
Left					
34. Neck Oblique Flexors Right					
Left					

Range—Check (✔) One

Date _____

RANGE OF MOTION EVALUATION

ZONE 4
Arms, Elbows, Wrists, and Hands

		Degree of Range of Motion	Red	Yellow	Green	Blue
35. Elbow Flexors	Right					
	Left					
36. Biceps	Right					
	Left					
37. Triceps	Right					
	Left					
38. Radio-Ulnar Supinators	Right					
	Left					
39. Radio-Ulnar Pronators	Right					
	Left					
40. Wrist Flex—Palms Down	Right					
	Left					
41. Wrist Flex—Palms Up	Right					
	Left					
42. Wrist Extensors	Right					
	Left					
43. Finger Flexors	Right					
	Left					
44. Finger Extensors	Right					
	Left					
45. Straight Finger Rotation		**No Range**				
46. Finger Webbing/Adductor		**No Range**				

Range—Check (✔) One

Date _____

RANGE OF MOTION EVALUATION

ZONE 5
Lower Legs, Ankles, and Feet

Range—Check (✔) One

		Degree of Range of Motion	Red	Yellow	Green	Blue
47. Soleus	Right					
	Left					
48. Achilles Tendon	Right					
	Left					
49. Gastrocnemius	Right					
	Left					
50. Tibialis Anterior	Right					
	Left					
51. Ankle Evertors	Right					
	Left					
52. Ankle Invertors	Right					
	Left					
53. Foot Pronators	Right					
	Left					
54. Foot Supinators	Right					
	Left					
55. Metatarsal Arch	Right					
	Left					
56. Toe Extensors	Right					
	Left					
57. Toe Flexors	Right					
	Left					
58. Big Toe Adductor		No Range				
59. Toe Webbing		No Range				

Date _____

Index

Abdominals, 10, 12, 28, 30, 40
Abductor:
  minimi digiti, 90
  in toes, 113
Achilles tendon:
  contracture, 220
  stretches for, 94–95
Aching, xxv, 211–212. *See also specific ailments*
Active-isolated stretching, generally:
  success of, xxv
  system described, xiv
  21-day guarantee, xv
Adductor(s):
  brevis, 18, 20, 36
  generally, 28, 30
  hallucis, 112
  longus, 18, 20, 36
  magnus, 18, 20, 36
  pollicis, 90
  in toes, 113
Aerobic instructor, credentials, 120
Aerobics/aerobic dancing, xxvi, 120–121
Aging process, impact of:
  bone strength, 208–209
  falls, 205–206
  flexibility and, 204–205, 209
  generally, 203–204
  joint problems, 206–207
  mental functioning, 209
  posture, 209
  sleep patterns, 207–208
Agonist, defined, 3

Amenorrhea, 124
Ankle, *see* Zone 5 (Lower Legs, Ankles, Feet)
  evertors, 100–101
  invertors, 102–103
  sprains, 131
Ankle-foot dorsal flexors, 92, 94, 96, 98
Antagonist, defined, 3
Anterior muscles, major, 5
Arches:
  metatarsal, 108–109
  strengthening exercises, xxvi–xxvii
Arms, *see* Zone 4 (Arms, Elbows, Wrists, Hands)
Artificial turf, 133
Asleep muscles, 212
Aspirin, xxvii–xxviii
Assistant, function of, xxxii, 7. *See also specific stretches*
Asthma, xxviii
Atherosclerosis, 210
Athlete, defined, xvi
Atrophy, xxi, xxv
Attitude changes, xxv

Baseball/softball, 121–122
Basketball, 122–123
Biathlons, 169–171
Biceps:
  brachii:
    generally, 50, 76, 78, 80, 82–83
    upper, 60
  generally, 78–79
Bleeding, prolonged, xxviii
Blood flow, xiv, xxii, xxviii

About the Authors

Jim and Phil Wharton

Nicknamed "The Mechanic" at the Olympic Games in Barcelona, Jim Wharton is known internationally for his ability to prepare and repair athletes so that they can perform at optimum levels to win. Recruited by a consortium of Olympic athletes and their coaches, Jim Wharton and his son and partner Phil worked extensively with members of the U.S. Track and Field Team and the U.S. Swim Team. In 1992, the United States returned from Barcelona with 30 medals in Track and Field and 27 medals in Swimming. Thirteen of those Olympic medals were around the necks of athletes who had enjoyed the Whartons' professional care.

The media focused attention on Jim and Phil Wharton in Barcelona. The growing demands placed on them by athletes all over the world convinced them that they needed to find a way to make their work and knowledge more available to athletes and sports enthusiasts—sharing their method just the way their mentor and teacher, Aaron Mattes, had shared it with them. Practicing from Maximum Performance International (http://www.aistretch.com/), their clinic in New York City, they continue to travel the world, teaching and lecturing.